Trauma Informed Su and Supervision for C Protection Professionals

This book presents a narrative approach to creating a supportive environment for health and human service practitioners who work with vulnerable children and their families – one of the most difficult and complex areas of practice.

People working in these environments are routinely exposed to violence and trauma and commonly experience symptoms of traumatic stress as a result. Traditionally, human service and health care service organisations have struggled to support practitioners who experience primary and secondary trauma in either a preventative context or post exposure. Using contemporary trauma theory, this book provides a trauma informed support and supervision framework for supervisors and managers of practitioners that recognises the uniqueness of the practice field, the diversity of practitioners who undertake the work and the diversity of contexts in which they work.

It will be required reading for all human service and health professionals, including social workers, psychologists and nurses, as well as teachers, counsellors and youth workers.

Fiona Oates is a social work–trained practitioner, consultant, educator and researcher with 20 years of experience working with vulnerable children and their families. Dr Oates has a strong interest in supporting the professional development and wellbeing needs of practitioners working in trauma-laden environments with an emphasis on child protection. Dr Oates has developed a model of support that is trauma informed and practitioner centered: the TISS model. The TISS model acknowledges the challenging occupational environment of practitioners that work with vulnerable children and has context-specific strategies embedded within. Dr Oates is based in Far North Queensland, Australia.

Trauma Informed Support and Supervision for Child Protection Professionals

A model for those working with children who have experienced trauma, abuse and neglect and their families

Fiona Oates

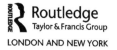

Routledge
Taylor & Francis Group

LONDON AND NEW YORK

First published 2023
by Routledge
4 Park Square, Milton Park, Abingdon, Oxon OX14 4RN

and by Routledge
605 Third Avenue, New York, NY 10158

Routledge is an imprint of the Taylor & Francis Group, an informa business

© 2023 Fiona Oates

British Library Cataloguing-in-Publication Data
A catalogue record for this book is available from the British Library

Library of Congress Cataloging-in-Publication Data
A catalog record for this book has been requested

ISBN: 978-0-367-45894-2 (hbk)
ISBN: 978-0-367-45895-9 (pbk)
ISBN: 978-1-003-02600-6 (ebk)

DOI: 10.4324/9781003026006

Typeset in NewBaskerville
by Apex CoVantage, LLC

I would like to dedicate this book to all the practitioners who are working or who have worked in this most challenging field, including my own teachers and mentors. You make a difference and you matter.

Contents

x *Contents*

Figures

Preface

Child protection work is one of the most rewarding and challenging vocations in the human, social and health services practice landscape. A manager of mine used to say that statutory child protection work was like any vice – the highs are very high, and the lows very, very low. As I have progressed through my 20-year career as a practitioner, researcher, educator and author this sentiment rings as true now as it did then. I have enormous respect for practitioners who choose to undertake child protection work as a vocation. It is quite incredible when beginning our professional journey into this area of work how quickly our ability to sit with the dreadfulness which is child abuse and neglect increases. I think it would be fair to say that almost every practitioner working in the area of child protection has told people they don't know at a party or non-work function what they do for a living and receive responses to the effect of, 'I don't know how you do that, I could never do that' or 'Wow, that must be so hard'. When I was a frontline practitioner, I found these conversations awkward and felt I never really had a satisfactory response. Now I see those occasions as reminders that the work professionals undertake in this area, although critically important, is extremely difficult and a vocation not suited to every human and social service worker. I would also like to give a special mention to those professionals who did not so much choose to work with vulnerable children and their families but have found themselves increasingly working with this cohort. As austerity measures continue to impact the delivery of social support services, particularly in Western countries, working with children and families where child protection concerns are present is a task increasingly falling on professionals outside of tertiary statutory child protection services and into universal and secondary services like health and education settings.

As a professional workforce, we are witness to the most horrific and unjust stories of violence, oppression and trauma experienced by the people we work with. We acknowledge that human brains are not designed to be saturated in the experience or persistent threat of violence. We further acknowledge that support that is trauma informed is the best evidence-based intervention to assist people to manage their traumatised brains as a measure to improve their wellbeing, functioning and overall quality of life. We ask a lot of the people we work with. We ask them to confront their complex histories of trauma and violence which are often underpinned by structural and societal disadvantage and oppression. We ask them to change a lifetime of maladaptive coping mechanisms in a short period of time. We ask this of people while the constant threat of losing their children either temporarily or permanently is endlessly present. Vulnerable children and their families need practitioners who have the skills and knowledge to guide them through their own experience of trauma and into a landscape that better meets the care and protective needs of children. They also need practitioners who have access to trauma informed support and supervision as a method of managing their own experiences of occupational traumatic stress.

Throughout the book are case studies that demonstrate the challenges encountered by practitioners, including line supervisors and managers, while working with vulnerable children and their families. These case studies are drawn from my own experience as a practitioner, supervisor, consultant, educator and researcher in the child welfare sector.

Introduction

Introduction

This book is written for professionals ranging from students to managers who in the course of their work have contact with vulnerable children and their families. My goal is to provide a conversational, easy-to-read, practical introduction to child protection work in traditional and non-traditional settings. Working with children who have experienced complex trauma is a highly specialised vocation requiring deep knowledge and a skill set responsive to the presenting needs of an individual. It also requires a great deal from the practitioners themselves, as working with people who have experienced complex trauma can be extremely taxing personally and requires careful management of one's own responses both in a professional setting with clients and in one's own personal life and space. The purpose of this book is to change the frame in which we see the wellbeing struggles of practitioners when working in this most difficult of human, social and health services practice. Normalising the experience of occupational trauma-related symptomology is critical and will support the creation and implementation of more effective and responsive support and supervision plans for practitioners.

Throughout the book, considerations for First Nations practitioners are included. The voices of First Nations practitioners who have participated in my own research are heard throughout. The support and supervision needs of First Nations peoples who undertake child protection work is a research focus of mine and is desperately under-researched.

The TISS (Trauma Informed Support and Supervision) framework presented in this book is underpinned by trauma informed practice principles – the same principles implemented by most contemporary workforces that interact with vulnerable children and their families.

DOI: 10.4324/9781003026006-1

By using trauma informed principles to support the wellbeing needs of the child protection workforce, it is anticipated that the blame culture that often blocks practitioners from seeking assistance will shift the deficit focus that underpins many practitioner wellbeing support models and programs to a more holistic, practitioner-centred evidence-based approach.

This book is divided into four chapters, about trauma, supervision, managers and organisations, and the final chapter, which introduces and discusses the application of the TISS model. The book has a scaffolded structure, meaning that core concepts are introduced and discussed with case examples used to demonstrate applicability in practice. The beginning chapters lay the foundational knowledge needed for readers to effectively engage with the TISS model outlined in the last section of the book.

This chapter introduces shared definitions of what constitutes child abuse and neglect, practice settings where practitioners engage with vulnerable children and their families and professional disciplines that work in this area. Also discussed is a brief outline of what supervision is and why supervision is important in the human and social services field.

Chapter One, Trauma, introduces the concept of trauma: what trauma is in a general sense and what trauma looks like in an occupational context. Primary, secondary and vicarious trauma symptomology are discussed as well as features of compassion fatigue and burnout. Organisational barriers to practitioners seeking support are addressed inclusive of the impact of not seeking support for occupational trauma symptomology on the practitioner, client and organisation. The prevention and treatment of occupational trauma is introduced, as is the concept of trauma informed work.

Chapter Two, Supervision, introduces the concept of supervision, what it is, common forms of supervision and the value it brings to professionals working with vulnerable children and their families. Supervision in an organisational context is discussed, as is the supervisory relationship. The chapter ends with the introduction and exploration of trauma informed supervision in a child welfare occupational context.

Chapter Three, Managers and Organisations, discusses the role of managers and line supervisors in an occupational context. The training and support needs of line supervisor and manager is discussed, as is the supervisory relationship from the perspective of the line supervisor or manager. Common challenges and dilemmas experienced by line supervisors and managers are outlined and discussed via the inclusion of case studies and vignettes. The impact of managerialism on the role of line supervisors and managers and their ability to provide support and supervision to their teams is discussed. Ending the chapter is a discussion about leadership and management in an organisational context and what a trauma informed, secure base leadership style might look like in practice.

The final chapter introduces the TISS framework. This chapter explores the central tenets of the TISS framework, including the creation of care teams around practitioners, identifying and mitigating threats to responsive support, as well as the underpinning principles of the framework. Throughout are practical examples of how the TISS framework could be applied in practice.

In this introductory chapter I introduce clear definitions of what constitutes child abuse and neglect in an Anglo-Western context. This is for two purposes. The first purpose is to educate readers who may be at the beginning of their studies, career or further professional development related to working with vulnerable children who have experienced abuse and neglect and their families. The second is to keep in the fore of the reader's mind the kinds of trauma children experience or are at risk of experiencing and by extension, that practitioners in this field are exposed to on a daily basis. Using generic terms creates the opportunity for those of us in the profession to not emotionally engage with the saturation of child abuse material we are exposed to on a daily basis while undertaking work with vulnerable children and their families. It also creates an environment more broadly for managers, funders or those outside of the organisation, like elements of the media, to not fully engage with what it is practitioners working in child protection manage as part of their roles.

What is child abuse and neglect?

Child abuse and neglect occurs in childhood and can be characterised as a single event or a prolonged period of linked or unlinked events. Harm can be interfamilial, that is, from within the family structure, or extrafamilial, outside the family structure, such as neighbours, teachers or coaches. Those perpetrating the harm can be adults or other children and peers. The settings in which child abuse or neglect occurs vary widely and can include the family home, the homes of extended family or family friends, houses of worship, educational settings, sporting or community groups and workplaces (older young people). Increasingly, environments accessed by children and young people via the internet are places where abuse can occur, such as chat type applications and gaming platforms.

There is some variation in the literature about what acts constitute child abuse and neglect. However, the general consensus is that child abuse and neglect can be grouped into four main subcategories, namely, physical abuse, emotional abuse, sexual abuse and neglect (Australian Institute of Family Studies, 2018). Of note is that the Canadian government includes exposure to domestic and family violence as a fifth stand-alone subcategory, as do other countries, like Australia and parts of the United Kingdom. In jurisdictions where this is not the case, like the United States and New Zealand, exposure to domestic and family violence is most commonly included under the emotional harm subcategory. I will now briefly outline what constitutes the most widely agreed-on definitions of those subcategories for the purpose of having a shared definition.

Physical abuse

Physical abuse harm is usually categorised as deliberate acts of physical aggression by others resulting in a traumatic response from the child involved. A child does not need to have physical injuries to be assessed as having experienced physical harm; the child's response to these situations is a key factor in assessing whether or not harm has occurred. The acts commonly agreed on as methods used to perpetrate physical harm include hitting, slapping, shaking, throwing, biting, burning and poisoning. Excessive discipline is also included in this harm category, however the definition of where physical discipline starts and where child abuse begins can vary widely between countries and contexts. Physical harm can also be experienced by children and young people as a result of an adult's inactions. These situations tend to unfold where caregiving adults are impaired by the problematic use of alcohol or other substances resulting in lack of supervision, as an example. Injuries to children that occur in an accidental context as a result of dysfunctional parental behaviour tend to be assessed to be in the emotional harm subcategory in many countries and are commonly referred to as harm caused by 'failure to protect'.

Sexual abuse

The sexual abuse harm category is clearly defined in the literature with agreement of what defines the sexual abuse of children across jurisdictions. Perpetrators of child sexual abuse can be adults or other children like siblings or peers, usually where there is a power imbalance. The acts that constitute child sexual abuse are wide and include penetration of a child in any way with a body part or other item, forcing a child to participate in sexual acts, exposing oneself to a child, exposing a child to sexual material like pornography and exploiting a child for one's own financial gain, prostitution as an example. Grooming is also considered in the sexual abuse harm category, although the definition can vary across jurisdictions and can sometimes be substantiated as emotional harm or neglect if the primary parent was aware of these behaviours and failed to act in a way that would secure the child's safety from the perpetrator.

Emotional abuse

Emotional harm and psychological harm are often used interchangeably in the literature regarding child abuse. What constitutes emotional harm of a child also varies widely across jurisdictions and is often context dependent. The statutory child protection agency in Queensland, Australia, defines emotional abuse to be when a 'child's social, emotional, cognitive or intellectual development is impaired or threatened' (DCYJMA, 2022). Some agreed-on acts that can result in emotional harm of a child are parental rejection and persistent threats of abandonment, hostility, scapegoating, sustained criticism and/or belittling. Other acts cited include educational or social isolation. As with the physical abuse harm category, the emphasis is on the impact to the child rather than the act itself.

The emotional harm subcategory can often accompany a practitioner's assessment of the primary reason for harm of a child. An example might be that a child has been physically injured as a result of domestic violence between their caregivers, however emotional harm may also be substantiated due to the child's witnessing of ongoing violence and threats to their internal sense of safety.

Neglect

There is consistency about some core caregiver actions and impacts on children that constitute neglect. These are when the basic necessities of life are withheld from a child, resulting in significant deficits to their health and wellbeing. Basic necessities of life are usually defined to be food, shelter, clothing, medical care and age-appropriate supervision. Similar to the emotional harm category, what constitutes neglect and under what circumstances can be heavily reliant on context. For example, if a parent is failing to provide adequate nutrition to their child but is residing in a refugee camp, for example, does this constitute neglect to the threshold of child abuse when the parent has no way of providing such things? Similarly, for populations in remote areas where access to health care can be limited, does the lack of provision to a child constitute neglect when access is problematic or not available? In both of these examples, the impact on children is great and at times could be life limiting, but how harm to the child is measured may vary between jurisdictions.

As mentioned, of note is that defining what constitutes child abuse and neglect is not always straightforward and is highly influenced by context – for example, children living is countries where war exists, or where there are limited legal protections. In acknowledgement of this I feel it appropriate to include an expanded definition of child abuse and neglect relied on by the World Health Organization (2006):

> All forms of physical and/or emotional ill-treatment, sexual abuse, neglect or negligent treatment or commercial or other exploitation, resulting in actual or potential harm to the child's health, survival, development or dignity in the context of a relationship of responsibility, trust or power.
>
> (p. 9)

There is agreement in the literature that child abuse and neglect concerns relate to children and young people aged 0 to 18 years of age. Some jurisdictions, for example Australia, allow for child protection concerns to be recorded in relation to unborn children.

Who works with children who have experienced abuse and neglect?

Many contemporary texts relating to child protection are based on practice in a statutory context, most often with involuntary clients. These texts also tend to be written by social work researchers, practitioners and academics. While acknowledging that these contemporary texts are highly relevant, statutory child protection agencies and those practitioners who work in that context are only some of the professionals who work with vulnerable children and their families. As mentioned earlier in this chapter, the kinds of settings where professionals are working with children and families where child protection concerns are present is widening. It is difficult to determine from the literature exactly why this has occurred; however, anecdotally practitioners believe that recent inquiries into the sexual abuse of children in institutions has lifted consciousness around child abuse and neglect. In addition, many Western countries have seen sustained cuts to social services designed to target at-risk families, moving the need into more universal services like health care and education. The rise of managerialism and its impact on social services is discussed in later chapters. I will now introduce the practice settings where professionals deliver services to vulnerable children and their families.

Statutory child protection

Statutory child protection services in Western countries are generally administered by the government, local, state or territory or federal government, and are underpinned by legislation. It is usually statutory child protection agencies that investigate allegations of harm occurring within a family unit. Statutory child protection agencies are also responsible for seeking custody or guardianship through the courts when parents are deemed unable to provide for the care and protective needs of their child/ren. When the state is awarded guardianship of a child, the state becomes in loco parentis, meaning it assumes all responsibilities that a parent might have, including financial. There are other custody arrangements where the state assumes a portion of in loco parentis responsibility, like decision making power over where a child may live or whom they have contact with, while some responsibilities remain with the parents, like decisions regarding medical care, for example.

Intensive parenting and family support services

These services tend to work with children and families who have been referred by a statutory authority where child protection concerns have been assessed to be present. These services are almost always voluntary and can include counselling, budgeting or financial literacy, parenting support or supported play groups. Many of these programs are funded by government with the goal of supporting families to address the child protection concerns present within their families and to reduce the likelihood of entry into the statutory child protection system.

Out-of-home care professionals

Children who are in the care of the state under care and protection orders in Western countries are referred to as 'looked-after children', or as living in 'out-of-home care', as examples in the practice literature. The scope of work undertaken by professionals in these settings is broad. Practitioners may work with families who wish to resume the care of their children or with children who have been in long-term care and require support transitioning into adulthood. Practitioners also work with foster, kinship and professional carers, supporting them to meet the needs of children in their care. The scope also includes, in some jurisdictions, adoption.

Residential care settings

Another form of out-of-home care is residential care. Children and young people living in residential care facilities tend to have more complex care and protective needs which often cannot be met in a traditional foster family setting. Children and young people living in residential care settings have often been exposed to significant amounts of trauma which may present as mental ill-health, alcohol or other substance misuse, a propensity for risk-taking behaviour and at times, violence towards themselves and others. Practitioners working in residential care settings experience persistent threats of violence as well as high levels of actual violence, including sexualised violence. Regulation of residential care settings varies widely across jurisdictions, as does the minimum qualification required of staff working within them.

Therapeutic intervention

This sub-category includes professionals who work in more traditional counselling or therapy settings with both child and adult clients as well as families in a family therapy context, as an example. Clients may be publicly or privately funded, voluntary or mandated.

Domestic and family violence services including sexual assault

This sub-category includes professionals working in women's shelters, domestic and family violence services that provide adult and child counselling services, telephone hotline and internet-based workers, and liaison staff within health settings where sexual assault matters are managed both medically and forensically for potential justice outcomes.

Youth services

Services provided to young people by organisations in the youth sector vary widely. However, youth are generally defined to be people of

12 to 25 years of age. Services could include access to drop-in spaces, emergency food relief, housing assistance, drug and alcohol support, support with legal matters, young parenting programs, employment assistance and improving access to education and training. Many youth services also have an advocacy role for the purpose of influencing government policy and program design.

Allied health professionals in health settings

For the purpose of this book, the term 'allied health workers' refers to nurses, doctors, dentists, social workers, occupational therapists, physiotherapists that work in general practice settings. Allied health professionals also work in, hospitals including accident and emergency departments, adult and child in-patient mental health facilities, community mental health services, sexual health and child and maternal health.

Justice workers

For the purposes of this chapter, justice workers encompass professionals working in courthouses, youth detention facilities and on multidisciplinary casework teams managing youth offenders in the community. The intersection between young people involved in the youth justice system and the experience of childhood abuse and neglect is well documented in the literature, but this nexus is seldom defined when it comes to program design and service delivery. Professionals working in adult correctional and other justice settings also manage matters pertaining to child abuse and neglect. Instances where this may occur may be through the collation of pre-sentence reports which outline an adult offender's history of child abuse, overview of matters where children have been the victims of crime or while visiting the home of clients who may be being supervised in the community. Professionals who access their clients in their own homes are often confronted with conditions where a notification to child protective services is warranted.

Disability support

Disability support work encompasses a broad range of practice types and settings. The professionals working in this area have a myriad of professional educational backgrounds ranging from degree-qualified allied health professionals right through to generalist support workers, some of whom work in positions where this is no minimum qualification requirement. Work with clients can include personal care and support to child or adult clients, engaging clients in community activities including social, assessment of functionality, care planning and case management. This work occurs in relations to clients living with all ranges of disability including psychiatric.

Legal professionals

Practice settings in this domain include the children's court, family court, criminal matters, and parole and sentence review boards. Professional groups include interpreters and other court liaison staff. Similar to justice professionals, law professionals are exposed to vast amounts of child abuse and neglect as part of their roles. Lawyers working with both child and adult clients are frequently exposed to detailed police interviews and other evidence like detailed medical reports. This group includes magistrates, judges and other court support staff, but again, this is a professional group seldom included in general literature relating to professionals who traditionally work with vulnerable children and their families.

Police and other emergency services

Emergency services workers in the context of this book refer to police and ambulance officers as well as firefighters and search-and-rescue professionals. Over the course of their work, emergency services workers enter the homes of vulnerable members of the community, including vulnerable children and their families. For the police, there are a number of protocols in place regarding when children are present during drug raids, domestic and family violence or other official police business. Although the literature is scarce, it does appear that police training regarding child abuse and neglect is not uniform across jurisdictions.

Teachers and other education staff

Teachers and education staff work in a number of settings, among them early childhood education inclusive of child care centres, primary and secondary school settings, as well as support staff who may work in homework clubs or youth group settings. In research undertaken by Hunt and Broadley (2020), a large number of educational professionals in Australia were studied, exploring experiences of identifying and responding to suspicions of child sexual abuse. Hunt and Broadley (2020) found that educational professionals experience many barriers to identifying and reporting child sexual abuse despite being mandated to do so, including a lack of specific training, uncertainty around what constitutes abuse and disillusionment with the statutory child protection authority.

Housing and homelessness service providers

Housing and homelessness services vary across jurisdictions. However, in summary, the housing and homelessness service delivery sector offers a wide range of services to vulnerable children and families who are, or are at risk of experiencing homelessness and/or housing instability. This practice domain is one that is often overlooked as a key practice area where professionals work with vulnerable children and young people who have experienced abuse or neglect in their families of origin. The link between homelessness and the experience of complex trauma is clear in the research literature. Children and families experience homelessness for a multitude of reasons; however, domestic and family violence (AIHW, 2014), parental experience of mental ill-health (Bromfield et al., 2012), problematic alcohol and other substance misuse (Foust et al., 2019) and circumstances related to poverty (O'Donnell et al., 2014) feature heavily in the literature. Children and young people who experience homelessness are more likely to have sporadic engagement or disengagement with education, health and other support services, often leading to suboptimal outcomes in adulthood (Foust et al., 2019; Parry et al., 2015).

Importance of recognising broad practice fields

It is important to recognise the broad and diverse practice settings professionals are working in. There is an assumption that statutory child protection practitioners work in organisations that, as per their policies and procedures, provide access to supervision. This is not always the case in other organisations, particularly those where traditional child protection work is undertaken, like in a hospital or legal setting. This leaves a large percentage of professionals who work with vulnerable children and their families without appropriate support or supervision. It also means that some professionals undertaking this work are in line management arrangements with supervisors who have never worked in child protection and may not have a deep understanding of the practice context or environment. I will elaborate on the importance of this throughout the book.

Chapter summary

In this chapter, a brief summary of the foundational knowledge of what constitutes child abuse and neglect was outlined. Who works with vulnerable children and families and in what practice settings was also briefly explored. In the next chapter, trauma will be explored, including what trauma is, how it affects those who experience it and what it looks like in an occupational context.

References

Australian Institute of Family Studies. (2018). *What is child abuse and neglect? CFCA resource sheet.* http://aifs.gov.au/cfca/publications/what-child-abuse-and-neglect

Australian Institute of Health and Welfare. (2014). *Australia's health 2014* (Australia's Health series no. 14. Cat. no. AUS 178). AIHW.

Bromfield, L., Lamont, L., Parker, R., & Horsfall, B. (2012). Issues for the safety and wellbeing of children in families with multiple and complex problems. *Child Family Community Australia, 33,* 1–25.

Department of Children, Youth Justice and Multicultural Affairs. (2022, January 5). *Protecting children.* Queensland Government. https://cyjma.qld.gov.au/protecting-children

Foust, R., Nghiem, H. T., Prindle, J., Hoonhout, J., McCroskey, J., & Putnam-Hornstein, E. (2019). Child protection involvement among homeless families. *Journal of Public Child Welfare, 14*(5), 518–530. doi:10.1080/15548732.2019.1651437

Hunt, S., & Broadley, K. (2020). Education professionals' role in identifying and reporting child sexual abuse: Untangling the maze. In I. Bryce & W. Petherick (Eds.), *Child sexual abuse* (pp. 391–419). Academic Press. https://doi.org/10.1016/B978-0-12-819434-8.00019-2.

O'Donnell, M., Varker, T., & Cash, R. (2014). The trauma and homelessness initiative. In M. A. Misio (Ed.), *Report prepared by the Australian Centre for post-traumatic mental health in collaboration with Sacred Heart.* Inner South Community Health and Vincent Care Victoria.

Parry, Y., Grant, J., & Burke, L. (2015). A scoping study: Children, policy and cultural shifts in homelessness services in South Australia: Are children still falling through the gaps? *Health & Social Care in the Community, 24*(5), e1–e10. doi:10.1111/hsc.12309

World Health Organization. (2006). *Preventing child maltreatment: A guide to taking action and generating evidence.* WHO. www.who.int/violence_injury_prevention/publications/violence/child_maltreatment/en/

1   Trauma

Introduction

In this chapter, the concept of trauma is discussed. It is important to have clear in our minds, as professionals who work with those who have experienced trauma, what it actually is. How trauma presents is critical to understand. This understanding allows us to identify its symptomology in the people we work with, which allows us to craft an effective, evidence-based intervention. This framework is the same framework that underpins the TISS model of support and supervision. Exposure to violence and trauma is an occupational inevitability. We must be able to identify symptomology of trauma in ourselves in order to craft an effective, evidence-based support intervention, that is, the same process as the interventions we craft for our clients. For those practitioners reading this who are also line supervisors or managers, it is important to have a clear understanding of trauma and its presenting symptomology in an occupational setting so that you can effectively support the practitioners you supervise.

What is trauma?

In a generalised sense, trauma is described as a normal physiological response to a single event or series of events that are extreme or threatening in nature (Haskell & Randall, 2009). The Substance Abuse and Mental Health Services Administration (SAMHSA) offers a succinct working definition of trauma, namely:

> Individual trauma results from an event, series of events or set of circumstances that is experienced by an individual as physically or emotionally harmful or life threatening and that has lasting

DOI: 10.4324/9781003026006-2

adverse effects on the individual's functioning and mental, physical, social, emotional or spiritual wellbeing.

(SAMHSA, 2014, p. 7)

The International Society for Traumatic Stress Studies (ISTSS) adds that traumatic events that lead a person to feel overwhelmed or unable to cope with the resulting negative emotions can be the events that lead to ongoing experiences of traumatic stress symptomology. ISTSS also state that events which are interpersonal or intentional in nature, including childhood abuse and neglect, tend to be responsible for a greater experience of adverse psychological outcomes (ISTSS, 2022).

What is occupational trauma?

Now that trauma has been summarised in a generalised sense, I now discuss in more detail what occupational trauma is and how it affects professionals working with vulnerable children and their families. Graham (2012) defines occupational trauma as 'the psychological effects of trauma directly attributable to occupational activity' (p. 25). There is agreement in the literature that although the scope of trauma exposure for individuals is narrowed to events occurring while undertaking one's occupational duties, the negative symptomology experienced is similar to trauma symptomology experienced by the general population (Graham, 2012; Rubino et al., 2009). Trauma-related effects are grouped into three key categories, namely psychological or somatic, physical and social (Behnke et al., 2020; Graham, 2012). Psychological or somatic effects include internalised shame, negative self-image and esteem, features of depression and anxiety and exhaustion emotionally (Rubino et al., 2009; Behnke et al., 2020; Oates, 2019). Effects attributed to physical impacts of trauma include insomnia and other sleep disturbances, nausea and other digestive complaints, fatigue and overall poorer health (Eidelson et al., 2003; McFarlane & Bryant, 2007; Pyevich et al., 2003). The social impacts were outlined in the literature to include negative disruptions in family life and other relationships, an increase in maladaptive coping strategies like alcohol and other substance misuse and withdrawal from social interactions (Graham, 2012; Oates, 2019; Rantanen et al., 2011).

Trauma exposure in child protection work, including the experience of primary trauma

Working with children who have experienced abuse and neglect comes with some occupational inevitabilities. Professionals who work in this area are frequently exposed to traumatic material and events in their workplaces, including exposure to physical, psychological and sexual harm of children. These situations can include witnessing distressing instances of abuse to children during hospital admissions, during interviews or through viewing photographic, audio or visual evidence. In addition to witnessing instances of abuse and neglect experienced by children, children and young people who experience trauma can present with a number of disturbing and confronting behaviours. These behaviours can include public self-harm, drug overdose, harm to animals, perpetration of harm against other vulnerable children and aggression towards their caregivers and protection workers. Child protection practitioners are often the ones who witness these events, an example of which is outlined by a practitioner:

> *He started smashing his face into the wall repeatedly and just screaming.*
> *By this stage, he was starting to bleed at the nose . . . there's blood going*
> *everywhere . . . the screaming was the scariest part. He's four. (Mary)*

For professionals working outside of traditional child protection settings, the kinds of material they are exposed to can vary. As an example, professionals working in a health setting like a hospital, a general practice office or an infant and maternal outreach program will be more likely to be exposed to the physical injuries or other presentations of child abuse and neglect and may be involved in the treatment of injuries resulting from physical or sexual harm as well as neglect. Professionals working in a justice setting like a legal practice or police setting will have access to detailed medical reports including photographs and transcripts of child victim statements. Educational professionals will be exposed to the behaviour that is often displayed by children who have experienced abuse or neglect. Anecdotally, professionals in these environments can have more difficulty coping with these instances as it only makes up a proportion of their day-to-day duties, not their entirety.

Primary trauma

The levels of exposure to traumatic material for professionals who work with vulnerable children and their families are extremely high. This is of course an occupational hazard; however, the way in which organisations and peers frame these incidents has historically been unhelpful. There is a reasonable amount of research literature that explores secondary and vicarious trauma, compassion fatigue and burnout. I will explore these concepts in more depth later in this chapter. There is, however, a dearth of literature that explores the primary trauma that practitioners in this field experience. Exposure to parental violence has been reported in the research literature as well as anecdotal practitioner feedback to be a common experience for professionals working with children who have experienced abuse and neglect. For the purpose of this book, references to violence within the workplace will include threats of violence, intimidation and other aggressive interactions as well as physical violence. In a large study of 590 practitioners conducted by Hunt et al. (2016), approximately half indicated that they had had negative experiences with aggressive parents and caregivers in the past 6 months. Of the practitioners studied, 61% indicated being threatened in the past 6 months and 32% stated they had been threatened 3 or more times in the same period. These acts of violence included physical assaults, being denied access to exits, death threats, bomb threats, threats to harm own children and pets as well as stalking and being spat at.

Participants in my own research outlined frequent experiences with client-initiated violence consistent with practitioners in Hunt et al's (2016) work. Following are three de-identified experiences of violence shared by practitioners:

> *I remember once me and another case worker actually had to lock ourselves in a room with another [child] client in the service because they [child client] were just going crazy and smashing the place and throwing chairs and threatening everybody. We're trying to ring the police on the phone in this room.* (Sarah)
>
> *It got to the point where he was standing in front of the back door preventing us from leaving. The police had to talk to him through the back door to convince him to let us out.* (Alice)
>
> *Went to do a [family] contact and was physically assaulted by the father, he shoved me into a [large hard object].* (Mary)

During my own career working in trauma-laden environments, I have supervised many professionals who work with children and families where child protection concerns are present across different practice settings. As such I have heard many accounts of the violence and trauma experienced by practitioners. I will now share de-identified examples:

> *I walked out of the office with a colleague for lunch – I had forgotten to take my ID tags off – a woman approached me, screamed that I was 'one of them', pointing to my office, and then pushed me really hard. I have never*

seen her before – I have no idea who she was – I was so shocked I couldn't move or say anything – everyone in the street was looking at me. (Ally)

I removed her baby from the hospital a few days after birth – the mother had a number of children already in care. Over the next couple of months, I would see her wherever I went. In the work carpark, at the supermarket, at my kid's sporting events, etc. I would get phone calls at all hours of the night. Then my family started receiving phone calls, we have a distinctive surname so I guess she just went through the phone book – she would tell them that she was a school friend of mine looking to reconnect. This was before the days of Facebook. This went on for months and months – she ended up being charged with stalking. It was a very difficult time. (Nora)

I was working in residential care and the sub-contracting agency had recently had its funding reduced by the child protection authority – this meant that there were times I would be on shift by myself. One of these times, one of the young men who lived there tried to sexually assault me – I got away, locked myself in the office and phoned the police – my manager said I should have been more attuned to my surroundings – they pretty much blamed me. I never went back.

(Linda)A young person I was working with had significant self-harming behaviour. One day they came into the reception area of our office – they were highly agitated due to a fight with a peer – they had a large kitchen knife and proceeded to aggressively cut open previously stitched self-harm injuries up their arms – I yelled for the receptionist to phone an ambulance while I tried to calm the young person down so they would give me the knife. (Rebecca)

The sharing of these incidents is purposeful. The purpose is to remind us that working in this field is traumatic and often occurs in an occupational context where the constant threat of violence is present. It is easy to minimise events like these when you work in an area where these events are commonplace. The minimisation of such events is a key factor in practitioners not seeking support when they need to and line supervisors and managers not being proactive in identifying staff who may be struggling with matters pertaining to their wellbeing.

There are, of course, more extreme examples of client violence towards professionals working in this area, such as workers who have been seriously injured, requiring hospitalisation, and even workers who have lost their lives as a result of client violence. However, while these incidents do occur, they are not common. Holding these extreme examples as the benchmark for practitioners being 'allowed' to be significantly affected by client threats and violence is not helpful and fosters a culture of minimisation.

Trauma symptomology experienced by child protection practitioners

As mentioned previously, the presenting symptomology of trauma is vast and can be difficult to identify in oneself and in colleagues. Practitioners in my own research described experiences of emotional symptomology and negative impacts on their wellbeing after prolonged exposure to trauma in the workplace. The symptoms described by participants included disrupted sleep including insomnia and nightmares, difficulty managing emotions, excessive crying, anger and rage, inability to focus and manage time and excessive questioning of their decision-making capability and effectiveness as a practitioner. Also described were doubts of self-worth, panic attacks and other symptomology consistent with anxiety and depression. Next are four experiences shared by participants which highlight the presentation of symptomology:

> *I'd be in tears going to work, in tears after work. (Sarah)*
>
> *I went to my doctor, because I was an absolute mess. I couldn't open the door [to my office], I was hiding away from people . . . I had developed severe depression and anxiety and that still, you know, I still get angry about it at times. (Matilda)*
>
> *I'd come home and lock myself in my room for two hours and cry before I could function. Having children, you can't do that. That distresses them. So that's when it was like that final straw. I can't continue like this. I can't do this. This is not worth maintaining an income but not being able to maintain your wellbeing. (Mary)*
>
> *[After a work-related incident] that affected me emotionally, I didn't care about the paperwork or what had to be done, it wasn't a priority anymore. I'd already failed with the emotional side of that child, that child blamed me for removal from his family. So, when things like that happened, I could not – I felt like I was – I couldn't do the job anymore. (Rosalyn)*

A number of practitioners in my study described feeling an overwhelming sense of isolation professionally as well as disconnection from their friends and families. Other tangible outcomes experienced by practitioners as a result of struggling with occupational trauma were absenteeism, decreased motivation and non-completion of work.

Secondary and vicarious trauma, compassion fatigue and burnout in child protection work

In addition to the primary trauma experienced by professionals who work with vulnerable children and their families, practitioners commonly experience other occupational specific traumas, namely, secondary and vicarious trauma, compassion fatigue and burnout. There is consensus in the literature that people who work in a trauma-laden environment with individuals who have experienced trauma are at much higher risk of developing symptoms of vicarious trauma than are people who do not (Bober & Regehr, 2005; Bride, 2007; Devilly et al., 2009; Harrison & Westwood, 2009; Jankoski, 2010). Exposure to secondary and vicarious trauma is discussed in the literature as an inherent part of working with children and their families where child protection concerns are present or where a child has experienced significant trauma (Geller et al., 2004; Levy & Poertner, 2014; Munro, 2010; Wise, 2017). Given that these sources of trauma so heavily affect practitioners working with child protection matters, I will now summarise them and how they can manifest in the workplace.

Secondary and vicarious trauma

Vicarious and secondary traumatisation are discussed interchangeably in the literature. Pearlman and Saakvitne (1995) originally defined vicarious traumatisation as 'the cumulative transformation in the inner experience of the therapist that comes about as a result of empathic engagement with the client's traumatic material' (p. 31). Williams et al. (2012) added to the definition provided by Pearlman and Saakvitne to argue that vicarious trauma presentation in workers is 'a shift in the internal experience and psychological wellbeing' (p. 134). Of vicarious trauma and how it presents for professionals working with people who have experienced trauma, Regehr (2018) states that 'vicarious trauma refers to changes in cognitive schemas regarding self, others, or the safety of the world, as a result of repeated exposure to the suffering of others' (p. 8). The symptomology of vicarious trauma in practitioners can be difficult to identify due to the broad range of symptomology and manifestations among those who experience it. Abassary and Goodrich (2014) described the behavioural indicators exhibited by professionals experiencing burnout as exhaustion 'accompanied by distress, reduced effectiveness, decreased motivation, as well as dysfunctional attitudes and behaviours at work' (p. 66). Regehr (2018) groups the symptomologies of vicarious trauma experienced by practitioners into three core areas, namely, intrusion, arousal and avoidance (p. 8). Regehr (2018) characterises the intrusion domain to include symptomologies like intrusive thoughts, sleep disturbances like nightmares and distress when recalling events that have been traumatic. Within the arousal domain, one could expect to experience hypervigilance, concentration difficulties, behavioural outbursts or interrupted sleep. Of the avoidance category, Regehr (2018) cites that practitioners may manage their distressing symptomology 'through numbing, detachment, loss of memory regarding a traumatic event, and/or efforts to avoid thoughts or stimuli that are reminiscent of the event' (p. 8).

Compassion fatigue and burnout

Compassion fatigue is defined in the literature to be a condition that results from an accumulation of secondary or vicarious trauma in the workplace where practitioners have not been able to adequately process these events or resolve resulting symptomology (Regehr, 2018). Symptoms can be physical and/or psychological in nature. Practitioners may experience post-traumatic stress type symptoms including features of anxiety and depression, difficulty maintaining relationships in both personal and professional life and a decrease in job satisfaction or professional purpose (Figley, 2012; Hinds & Giardino, 2020). Behavioural indicators may include irritability, negativity, lower levels of concentration, persistent tiredness, depersonalisation or minimisation of suffering, both in a general sense as well as in regard to clients (Berzoff & Kita, 2010; Geoffrion et al., 2015).

The experience of compassion fatigue by practitioners can have a negative impact on clients. Compassion fatigue is characterised in the literature as involving a process whereby practitioners can become desensitised to the experiences of clients and their need, which can impair their ability to make sound evidence-based decisions, increasing the likelihood of mistakes (Figley, 2012; Hinds & Giardino, 2020; Regehr, 2018). These outcomes can result from a practitioner's preoccupation with the traumatic events that were the impetus for the onset of symptoms, persistent intrusive thoughts, hypervigilance or a sense of dread when faced with difficult material or clients leading to avoidance (Geoffrion et al., 2015).

Burnout

Burnout and compassion fatigue are often used interchangeably in the literature, mostly due to the similar symptomologies used to define both. The literature outlines that the symptomology experienced as result of both conditions include emotional and physical exhaustion, reduced job satisfaction, anxiety and depression as well as a decreased capacity for empathy (Figley, 2012; Hinds & Giardino, 2020; Regehr, 2018).

While the phenomenon of burnout can occur in any profession, McFadden (2020) argues that child protection professionals are at increased risk due to the inherent nature of the work and the occupational environment that work occurs in. In addition to constant exposure to traumatic material and events, professionals working in the area of child protection contend with additional stressors including unrealistic workloads, burdensome paperwork such as preparations for court matters, austerity measures limiting quality interventions, onerous media attention and negative perceptions by the public, all within an environment that is chronically under-resourced and under-staffed (Geoffrion et al., 2015; Hunt et al., 2016; McFadden, 2020; Regehr, 2018).

Other sources of trauma relevant to child protection practitioners and barriers to seeking assistance

Practitioners are often reticent to disclose that they are experiencing symptoms of vicarious trauma for fear of being viewed as deficient in some way (Hunt et al., 2016; Oates, 2019; Zerubavel & Wright, 2012). Pearlman (1995) argued with this sentiment and wrote that vicarious traumatisation is not a 'reflection of inadequacy on the part of the [practitioner] . . . it is best conceptualised as an occupational hazard' (p. 52). However, despite Pearlman's (1995) view that the experience of traumatic stress in those who work in trauma-laden environments is inevitable and should be considered as an occupational hazard, the literature suggests that child protection agencies struggle to manage the presentation of vicarious trauma and other trauma-based mental health concerns among practitioners (Goddard & Hunt, 2011; Littlechild, 2005), and that individual workers are often expected to manage their own wellbeing (Lewig & McLean, 2016).

In my own research, practitioners identified workplace culture as a barrier for them seeking assistance. Many practitioners shared that they had been, and in some cases still would be, reluctant to seek support, especially from direct line supervisors. These research participants described a workplace culture that does not allow workers to speak openly about experiencing symptoms of traumatic stress. Many participants believed the clear message was that, if a worker was not coping, they were incompetent:

> *There was almost a culture of if you say you're not coping, then you immediately become incompetent and you're immediately treated as being incompetent . . . basically, 'If you guys can't cope, maybe you should work*

somewhere else'. So it's almost like you don't want to speak up then because people think you can't do your job properly. (Mary)

 I guess in some respects it's frowned upon, it's almost like, you know, 'Oh, get over yourself', you know, 'If you want to work in this place, you need to harden up'. (Matilda)

 They would say, 'Do you think that's really something you should be talking about around the office? Aren't you worried that you'll lose your job?'. (Alice)

Additionally, some participants stated that, if a worker was experiencing symptoms of traumatic stress, they were not considered suitable for child protection work:

 I'm being told, 'Maybe you're not suited to your role'. I've been here [number] years, but okay, whatever. (Sarah)

 I went and saw the manager about it and she said, 'Yeah, well, maybe child [protection] work isn't for you – maybe you could work in projects or do a different job somewhere else'. (Rosalyn)

Reticence to seek support for occupational traumatic stress symptomology due to the fear of receiving a negative response is consistent with Hunt et al.'s (2016) mixed-methods study of child protection workers and their experiences of organisational and management response after an incident with hostile parents. Hunt et al. (2016) found that an organisational response that emphasised exposure to violence as part of the job and that arising symptomology was a deficit within the worker to be common. Participants in that study shared that the clear message from the organisation was for practitioners to 'improve their stamina and resilience' (Hunt et al., 2016, p. 14).

A number of studies (Hunt et al., 2016; Littlechild, 2005; Oates, 2019) have recommended that a systems review of organisations, particularly statutory organisations, be undertaken to identify the cultural and structural deficits that act as barriers to supporting practitioners affected by traumatic stress–related symptomology. However, there is a dearth of literature regarding whether these recommendations have been implemented and if so, what impact they have had. The role of line managers and organisations in managing practitioner wellbeing will be discussed in subsequent chapters.

Racism as trauma: considerations for First Nations practitioners

As previously mentioned, my doctoral research explored the experiences of Aboriginal and Torres Strait Islander child protection practitioners in Australia. At the time the study was undertaken, there was a dearth of research literature about what the unique needs of Aboriginal and/or Torres Strait Islander practitioners would be in the child protection workplace given their historical experience of state-sanctioned forced child removal. Indigenous children and families are grossly over-represented in all parts of the child protection continuum in Australia. However, Australia is not unique in this respect. First Nations children are disproportionately represented in child protection systems across jurisdictions and where the forced removal of children was a feature of colonisation like Canada, the United States and New Zealand.

In both an Australian and international context, there is agreement in the literature that there exists a clear connection between colonisation practices, the historical forced removal of children and other racially discriminatory social policy and the social issues affecting First Nations communities in a contemporary context (Atkinson, 2002; Bennett, 2013; Bessarab & Crawford, 2013; Sherwood, 2013). The disproportionate representation of First Nations children and families requiring the intervention of statutory child protective authorities is a demonstration of this nexus (Atkinson, 2002; Bennett, 2013; Menzies & Gilbert, 2013). Researchers, academics and practitioners have argued that the deep trauma experienced by First Nations communities where forced child removal was a feature of colonisation manifests contemporarily as parental maladaptive coping strategies and behaviours that would likely cause children and families to come to the attention of child protective authorities (Atkinson, 2002; Herring et al., 2013; King et al., 2009).

Many jurisdictions have increased recruitment of First Nations practitioners as a strategy to address the disproportionate representation of First Nations children and families requiring child protection services (Oates, 2020). Many complexities exist for First Nations practitioners who wish to undertake child protection work. One of these complexities is the central role the social work profession had in the forced removal of First Nations children from their families and communities. Indigenous Australian social work academic Bennett (2013) describes that at the time social work was an 'instrument of social control' (p. 19) and that social workers were 'participants in the process of dispossession and oppression' of Aboriginal people and communities (p. 20). Many Aboriginal and Torres Strait Islander people and communities have a deep sense of suspicion and distrust of social workers related to the role they played in the state-sanctioned forced removal of Indigenous children (Gilbert, 1993; Harms et al., 2011). Contemporarily, this is of particular relevance when considering what role Aboriginal and Torres Strait Islander practitioners in the child protection service system have and what their experiences might be in this context. Given the negative and racially discriminatory history (although some First Nations researchers and academics would argue it is still current) of First Nations people with child protection authorities, it is necessary to explore what the support needs of First Nations practitioners might be as they enter the child protection workforce.

My study found that First Nations practitioners overall had a deep desire to work within their communities. Many cited that helping others, particularly children, was a core cultural value and therefore central to their identity. Undertaking child protection work was a source of pride for practitioners, but their families had mixed feelings about their work in the child protection system. Practitioners cited that the negative reactions were out of concern for their wellbeing but also due to the historical experiences their communities have had with child protective authorities, with some expressing a sense of betrayal that their family member would go and work for 'the welfare'. Many practitioners in the study expressed conflict within themselves for the same reason. A number of participants described times when they experienced adverse emotional reactions when undertaking work that in some way triggered either their personal history or their family's history of forced child removal and resulting trauma.

In addition to occupational trauma triggering previous personal experiences of trauma rooted in the colonial practice of forced child removal, a number of practitioners experienced frequent occurrences of racism within their places of work. Practitioners shared a number of incidents of overt racism perpetrated by their colleagues. These incidents often took place in shared open-plan workspaces:

> This is somebody who had made references about, 'Well, these darkie kids are lucky to be in care because then they get food', or, 'At least the darkies will get to go to school every day over here', and things like that – she actually used the term 'darkie'. (Mary)
>
> What was the other really doozy one that we had? I was shocked. 'All black men have gonorrhoea'. That was a pearler. (Sarah)
>
> 'That just shows that blacks don't love their kids as much as other people do' [in relation to Torres Strait Islander traditional adoption practices]. (Sarah)
>
> 'All black kids have scabies'. I said, 'So, my kids are black. Do they have scabies?' 'Your kids are lovely. No, no, not you. You're different', she goes. 'You keep your kids clean'. (Mary)

Some of the instigators of these incidents were managers or senior members of staff:

> *Manager would never address it. Manager let it – I'll be blunt, she – the person led it. (Isabella)*
> *The team leaders are the prime offenders. (Sarah)*

Practitioners also described experiencing racism in relation to their appearance:

> '*You really don't look Aboriginal . . . it's lucky you're white enough that people don't know'. (Mary)*

Herring et al. (2013) argued that 'racism remains part of the day-to-day experience, debilitating our people, denying us the right to live and move about with ease in our own country, compounding the low self-esteem and shame that many people carry' (p. 108). According to Bryant-Davis and Ocampo (2005), negative emotional responses to experiencing racism 'fit the standard definition of trauma' (p. 574). Lowe et al. (2012) conducted a qualitative study into racism as a source of trauma, and concluded that participants who experience racism also experience trauma symptomology. Lowe et al. (2012) outlined that participant experiences were 'similar to trauma responses as described in the *Diagnostic and Statistical Manual of Mental Disorders*' (p. 195).

During this research I found that First Nations practitioners who work with children and families where child protection concerns are present experience the same level of exposure to occupational trauma as their non-Indigenous colleagues. However, their frequent experience of racism in the workplace is an additional source of trauma that needs to be addressed in support and supervision planning with First Nations staff.

Impacts of occupational trauma on practitioners, organisations and service delivery

In the literature, the impacts of practitioners experiencing traumatic stress unsupported are grouped into three main categories: impact on the practitioners (Hunt et al., 2016; Oates, 2019; Whinghter et al., 2008); impact on service delivery to clients (Hecht & Boies, 2009; Hunt et al., 2016; Regehr, 2018); and impact on the organisation

(Graham, 2012; Regehr, 2018). These three key categories will now be explored.

Impact on the practitioner

There is a moderate amount of research literature that explores the symptomology of occupational traumatic stress experienced by professionals working with children and families where child protection concerns are present. The impacts of these experiences are cited in the literature as a decrease in job satisfaction and performance (Hunt et al., 2016; Whinghter et al., 2008), poor self-esteem and self-image (Oates, 2019; Regehr, 2018), inability to connect with relationships both personal and professional (Oates, 2019), as well as symptomology consistent with anxiety and depression including formation of maladaptive coping strategies like an increase in alcohol and other substance use (Hunt et al., 2016; Graham, 2012; Oates, 2019; Regehr, 2018).

Practitioners in my own research described a deep sense of loss and failure after they left their roles in child protection. For many, undertaking child protection work was as much a part of their identity as it was a professional vocation. Many expressed grief of losing parts of their professional identity as well as workplace relationships. Interestingly, some practitioners reflected on their feeling that the loss of relationships and professional identity that occurred when they left their positions was worse than the original trauma or series of traumas that were the impetus for them leaving in the first place (Oates, 2019).

While a moderate amount of literature exists regarding the symptomology experienced by practitioners as a result of occupational traumatic stress, there is a dearth of research related to how these symptoms manifest, or resolve, longitudinally. Practitioners in my own research described some of their occupational traumatic stress symptomology to be ongoing even after they left their positions in child protection.

> *I was like I need to go and get help. That's when I really started to deal with the trauma that I have been through with [statutory child protection agency]. That was the first time, after two years [after leaving]. (Mary)*
>
> *The first time I had to go out to my old office for a meeting, I had a panic attack. Yeah, it was really, really difficult. Yeah, it's just whenever I talk about it, like I am now, I get that thumping feeling in my gut. (Matilda)*

Impact on client service delivery

The literature suggests that the impact on the quality of service delivery to clients as a result of unsupported practitioner experience of traumatic stress may be significant. Factors that may negatively affect service delivery to vulnerable clients include increased practitioner absenteeism (Parks & Steelman, 2008) and an impaired ability to manage the demands of their workload (Hecht & Boies, 2009; Oates, 2019), including their ability to make sound decisions (Regehr, 2018). Regehr (2018) has written extensively on how exposure to occupational trauma affects a practitioner's decision making capacity. Regehr (2018) states that

> professional decision making can be affected by both acute stress related to the current situation and traumatic stress responses to previous encounters. Individuals in acutely stressful situations may experience selective attention, focusing particularly on threat stimuli with limited ability to consider other factors. Acute stress impacts computational capacity, requiring individuals to rely more heavily on heuristics as deliberative cognitive processing and decision-making capacities are constricted.
>
> (pp. 13–14)

The sustained experience of traumatic stress can also impair memory. LeBlanc (2009) writes that a person's experience of acute stress can affect memory and reduce their ability to 'retrieve, store, consolidate and manipulate information (pp. 13–14).

Professionals who work with vulnerable children and their families work with the most vulnerable and complex client group. Working with children who have experienced trauma, and their families, requires a specialist knowledge base and skill set which reflect the complexities of the work. Practitioners carrying an impaired ability to make clear evidence-based decisions in relation to the safety of vulnerable children due to unsupported occupational traumatic stress symptomology is of great concern. Studies by Briggs et al. (2004), Ferguson (2011) and Hunt et al. (2016) indicate that when practitioners don't have strong professional support to manage occupational traumatic stress related symptomology, they could inadvertently put vulnerable children and families at risk. A study by Hunt et al. (2016) of 423 child protection practitioners found that 42% believed that the quality of their care and protection assessments were compromised because of a lack of adequate support and supervision. Briggs et al.

(2004) have argued that deficient provision of supervision to child protection practitioners leads to potential neglect of children's safety. Briggs et al. (2004) wrote that

> this situation could result in the rights and needs of abused children being ignored due to a loss of productivity, increased fear, loss of commitment and turnover of professionals in the field. It also heralds the need for attention to be paid to the mental health of professionals engaged in child protection.
>
> (p. 5)

Impact on the organisation

Impacts on organisations that employ professionals to work with children and families where child protection concerns are present can be wide ranging. The literature reports that the financial cost to organisations of unsupported practitioner experience of occupational traumatic stress include productivity loss affecting contractual arrangements (Kaminski, 2001), reputational damage due to poor work with clients or partner agencies including the ability to recruit staff (Whinghter et al., 2008), financial loss due to work-related injury claims (Searle, 2008) or negligence litigation from clients (Dollard et al., 2007), and the financial burden of constantly recruiting and training new staff due to inability to retain experienced practitioners.

The literature does indicate that the majority of the predicted impacts to organisations due to practitioner experience of unsupported occupational traumatic stress are financial in nature. However, the majority of organisations that employ professionals to work with vulnerable children and their families are government operated or government funded, resulting in the unplanned re-direction of public money away from essential services.

The treatment of trauma

Now that we have looked at what trauma is in a generalised and child protection occupational specific context, I will now briefly outline current thinking related to the treatment of trauma once it has occurred. As previously outlined, trauma is a normal reaction to an abnormal set of circumstances and is experienced as a persistent threat either real or perceived (Dickson, 2017; Regehr, 2018). The experience of trauma presents as a complex mix of physiological, psychological, and environmental elements (Regehr, 2018). Therefore, treatment for traumatic stress–related symptomology must address all of these elements to be successful. Assessing need and implementing interventions to meet presenting needs is a core skill set for any professional working with vulnerable children and families in any setting. However, when it comes to our own experience of occupational trauma, the process seems less straightforward.

There is a difference between trauma experienced in the general community and trauma experienced in an occupational setting. When the workplace is the source of one's trauma, it is the workplace that needs to become a place of safety. This is a key element and one that is often overlooked. When we liken this to a client's experience of trauma, the removal of the trauma and the creation of safety underpins our interventions. When the source of trauma cannot be removed, like a person's place of work or a person's profession, then other strategies are required.

Regehr (2018) advocates that organisations that employ practitioners in trauma-laden environments should have strategies to mitigate risks to practitioners but also to be part of the solution post-exposure. Regehr (2018) argues that organisations need to 'take responsibility for reducing exposure to the extent possible, for mitigating the impacts of stress and trauma exposure, and for providing services when individual social workers are suffering' (p. 16). To highlight the critical role organisations have in supporting practitioners to manage occupational traumatic stress–related symptomology, I will now briefly discuss what is referred to in the literature as the dosage-response relationship.

Dosage-response relationship

The dosage-response relationship is a term used to describe the correlation, or not, between the amount of trauma experienced and the likelihood of a person experiencing ongoing traumatic stress–type symptomology as a result. There are contradictory findings in the literature about whether there is a strong correlation between the two. Meyer et al. (2012) found in their study with firefighters no correlation between frequency of exposure and experience of traumatic stress symptomology. Meyer et al. (2012) did, however, find that factors like self-blame and perceived social and organisational support were more accurate predictors of ongoing clinically significant symptomology. Similarly, Regehr (2018) found in relation to social workers' exposure to trauma while undertaking their occupational duties that the nature of the trauma was not a predictor of ongoing traumatic stress symptomology but rather a 'complex interaction between the individual, the organisation, and the societal environment' to be a more definitive measurement (p. 15). Conversely, Behnke et al. (2020) found in a review of multiple studies exploring the dosage-response connection that the higher the number of traumatic incidents experienced by 'trauma-exposed' professions like emergency services personnel, the more likely the development of traumatic stress symptomology(p. 2). Behnke et al. (2020) further found that a history of childhood maltreatment was a significant factor that may predispose people working in trauma–exposed professions to ongoing traumatic stress symptomologies while undertaking occupational duties. Meyer et al. (2012) have hypothesised that the conflicting research outcomes in the literature may be a result of the research methodology chosen or the inconsistent application of said research methodologies within those studies.

Despite conflicting research findings regarding the dosage-response relationship, there is some common agreement in relation to factors that may lead to positive resolution of trauma-related stress symptomologies for practitioners. These factors include perceived social support and connection and satisfaction in the role and workplace. There is research literature that suggests that external environmental factors like an empathetic work environment including an attuned supervisor, a manageable workload and supervisory and peer support are more likely to result in the resolution of traumatic stress symptomologies over a longer period (McFadden et al., 2015; Regehr, 2018). These findings are significant as they support that what happens after a traumatic event may be more significant than the individual circumstances present for a person prior to a traumatic event taking place.

The resilience myth

The treatment of occupational trauma in the literature relevant to professionals who work with vulnerable children and their families tends to focus largely on the resilience of the individual practitioner. While studies show that resilience is a factor when predicting future longer-term struggles with occupational traumatic stress symptomology, it is not the only factor and is certainly not the 'silver bullet' to address issues pertaining to retention and job satisfaction in the child protection workforce.

Building resilience as part of professional identity relies on a full acknowledgement of the risks posed to practitioners working in this area. Without full acknowledgement, strategies implemented to build resilience within the workforce will not be effective. Strategies that support the internalising of occupational traumatic stress symptomologies by practitioners as a failure in their ability to have and maintain resilience is not an appropriate response by organisations, line managers or peers.

As presented earlier in this chapter, in my own research, being labelled as incompetent or not being suited to do child protection work when experiencing traumatic stress–related symptomology was identified as the strongest barrier for practitioners seeking timely support. Having stated that, practitioner resilience is not a silver bullet, but it is an important element when discussing supporting practitioners with occupational traumatic stress symptomology. I will discuss the notion of practitioner resilience in more detail over subsequent chapters.

What is 'trauma informed' as a general concept?

Trauma informed client-based interventions have become ubiquitous over the past decade. In nearly every area of human, social and health service practice, trauma informed practices have been adopted as the set of principles that underpin organisational service delivery with clients. Wall et al. (2016) describe trauma informed care in its simplest form to be 'a framework for human service delivery that is based on knowledge and understanding of how trauma affects people's lives and their service needs' (p. 9).

The literature outlines that there are six core principles of trauma informed care. These six principles are: safety; trustworthiness and transparency; peer support; collaboration and mutuality; empowerment including client voice and choice; and cultural, historical and gender issues and context (Harris & Fallot, 2001; SAMHSA, 2014). A trauma informed practitioner working with people who have experienced trauma would holistically consider a person's circumstances and craft an effective intervention accordingly. Trauma informed interventions with vulnerable children and their families must include an acknowledgement by the practitioner that welfare and health, including social and emotional health settings, are often triggers for people, increasing the potential for clients to be re-traumatised (Kezelman & Stavropoulos, 2012). Viewing the needs of clients in the context of their trauma history is consistent with a trauma informed approach (Knight, 2015).

The concept of trauma informed organisations or systems also features heavily in the literature. Whether it be trauma informed interventions for clients who have experienced trauma or trauma informed organisational operations, the overall goal is the same, namely, to not further traumatise people who are either serviced by or employed within these programs. SAMHSA (2014) defines a trauma informed approach to service delivery as follows:

> A program, organisation or system that is trauma informed real-ises the widespread impact of trauma and understands potential paths for recovery; recognises the signs and symptoms of trauma in clients, families, staff and others involved with the system and responds by fully integrating knowledge about trauma into policies, procedures and practices and seeks to actively resist re-traumatisation.
>
> (p. 9)

SAMHSA (2014) outlined that any organisation wishing to implement a trauma informed framework for service delivery must be under-pinned by four key elements: realisation, recognition, response and resist (commonly referred to in the literature as the four Rs). Wall et al. (2016, p. 9) summarise the four Rs as:

1. *Realisation* at all levels of an organisation or system about trauma and its impacts on individuals, families and communities;
2. *Recognition* of the signs of trauma;
3. *Response* – a program, organisation or system responds by apply-ing the principles of a trauma informed approach; and
4. *Resist* re-traumatisation of clients as well as staff.

This is a very brief summary of what trauma informed frameworks are. I will discuss the concept of trauma informed interventions as they relate to practitioners who work with vulnerable children and their families in more detail in the next chapter.

Chapter summary

In this chapter I have discussed what trauma is and how it may present, including common symptomology, in a general context. The chapter then moved to outlining occupational trauma and practitioner expo-sure to trauma in an occupational context. Practitioner experience of primary trauma as well as secondary and vicarious trauma and compas-sion fatigue are also outlined and discussed. The experience of racism in an occupational context was introduced as an additional source of trauma for First Nations practitioners. The impacts of occupational trauma on practitioners, clients and organisations was discussed, as were commonly accepted methods of treatment, including trauma informed interventions.

Reflective questions for practice

1. How do you think your own experience of trauma affects you professionally?
2. Thinking about your own experience of occupational trauma, what do you think would assist you, including organisationally, to move through distressing symptomology?

References

Abassary, C., & Goodrich, K. M. (2014). Attending to crisis-based supervision for counselors: The CARE model of crisis-based supervision. *The Clinical Supervisor, 33*(1), 63–81. doi:10.1080/07325223.2014.918006

Atkinson, J. (2002). *Trauma tails recreating song lines: The transgenerational effects of trauma in Indigenous Australia.* Spinifex Press.

Behnke, A., Rojas, R., Karabatsiakis, A., & Kolassa, I. (2020). Childhood maltreatment compromises resilience against occupational trauma exposure: A retrospective study among emergency medical service personnel. *Child Abuse & Neglect, 99*, 104248–104248. doi:10.1016/j.chiabu.2019.104248

Bennett, B. (2013). The importance of aboriginal and Torres Strait Islander history for social work students and graduates. In B. Bennett, S. Green, S. Gilbert, & D. Bessarab (Eds.), *Our voices: Aboriginal and Torres Strait Islander social work* (pp. 1–25). Palgrave Macmillan.

Berzoff, J., & Kita, E. (2010). Compassion fatigue and countertransference: Two different concepts. *Clinical Social Work Journal, 38*(3), 341–349. doi:10.1007/s10615-010-0271-8

Bessarab, D., & Crawford, F. (2013). Trauma, grief and loss: The vulnerability of Aboriginal families in the child protection system. In B. Bennett, S. Green, S. Gilbert, & D. Bessarab (Eds.), *Our voices: Aboriginal and Torres Strait Islander social work* (pp. 93–109). Palgrave Macmillan.

Bober, T., & Regehr, C. (2005). Strategies for reducing secondary or vicarious trauma: Do they work? *Brief Treatment and Crisis Intervention, 6*(1), 1–9. doi:10.1093/brief-treatment/mhj001

Bride, B. (2007). Prevalence of secondary traumatic stress among social workers. *Social Work, 52*(1), 63–70. doi:10.1093/sw/52.1.63

Briggs, F., Broadhurst, D., & Hawkins, R. (2004). Violence, threats and intimidation in the lives of professionals whose work involves children. *Trends and Issues in Crime and Criminal Justice, 273*, 1–6.

Bryant-Davis, T., & Ocampo, C. (2005). The trauma of racism: Implications for counseling, research, and education. *The Counseling Psychologist, 33*(4), 574–578. doi:10.1177/0011000005276581

Devilly, G., Wright, R., & Varker, T. (2009). Vicarious trauma, secondary traumatic stress or simply burnout? Effect of trauma therapy on mental health professionals. *Australasian Psychiatry, 43*(4), 373–385. doi:10.1080/00048670902721079

Dickson, M. (2017). *What does trauma informed mean? Grappling with the challenge.* http://professionals.childhood.org.au/prosody/2017/11/what-does-trauma informed-mean/

Dollard, M., LaMontagne, A., Caulfield, N., Blewett, V., & Shaw, A. (2007). Job stress in the Australian and international health and community services sector: A review of the literature. *International Journal of Stress Management, 14*(4), 417–445. doi:10.1037/1072-5245.14.4.417

Eidelson, R., D'Alessio, G., & Eidelson, J. (2003). The impact of September 11 on psychologists. *Professional Psychology, Research and Practice, 34*(2), 144–150. doi:10.1037/0735-7028.34.2.144

Ferguson, H. (2011). *Child protection practice.* Palgrave Macmillan.

Figley, C. (Ed.). (2012). Compassion fatigue. In *Encyclopedia of trauma: An interdisciplinary guide.* Sage. doi.org/10.4135/9781452218595.

Geller, J., Madsen, L., & Ohrenstein, L. (2004). Secondary trauma: A team approach. *Clinical Social Work Journal, 32*(4), 415–430. doi:10.1007/s10615-004-0540-5

Geoffrion, S., Morselli, C., & Guay, S. (2015 [2016]). Rethinking compassion fatigue through the lens of professional identity: The case of child-protection workers. *Trauma, Violence & Abuse, 17*(3), 270–283. doi:10.1177/1524838015584362

Gilbert, S. (1993). The effects of colonisation on Aboriginal families: Issues and strategies for child welfare policies. In J. Mason (Ed.), *Child welfare policy: Critical Australian perspectives.* Hale and Iremonger.

Goddard, C., & Hunt, S. (2011). The complexities of caring for child protection workers: The contexts of practice and supervision. *Journal of Social Work Practice, 25*(4), 413–432. doi:10.1080/02650533.2011.626644

Graham, J. (2012). Cognitive behavioural therapy for occupational trauma: A systematic literature review exploring the effects of occupational trauma and the existing CBT support pathways and interventions for staff working within mental healthcare including allied professions. *Cognitive Behaviour Therapist, 5*(1), 24–45. doi:10.1017/S1754470X12000025

Harms, L., Middleton, J., Whyte, J., Anderson, I., Clarke, A., Sloan, J., . . . Smith, M. (2011). Social work with aboriginal clients: Perspectives on educational preparation and practice. *Australian Social Work, 64*(2), 156–168. doi:10.1080/0312407X.2011.577184

Harris, M., & Fallot, R. (2001). Envisioning a trauma informed service system: A vital paradigm shift. *New Directions for Mental Health Services, 89*, 3–22. doi:10.1002/yd.23320018903

Harrison, R., & Westwood, M. (2009). Preventing vicarious traumatization of mental health therapists: Identifying protective practices. *Psychotherapy:*

Theory, Research, Practice, Training, 46(2), 203–219. doi:10.1037/a00 16081

Haskell, L., & Randall, M. (2009). Disrupted attachments: A social context complex trauma framework and the lives of aboriginal peoples in Canada. *Journal of Aboriginal Health, 5*(3), 48.

Hecht, T., & Boies, K. (2009). Structure and correlates of spillover from nonwork to work: An examination of nonwork activities, well-being, and work outcomes. *Journal of Occupational Health Psychology, 14*(4), 414–426. doi:10.1037/a0015981

Herring, S., Spangaro, J., Lauw, M., & McNamara, L. (2013). The intersection of trauma, racism, and cultural competence in effective work with Aboriginal people: Waiting for trust. *Australian Social Work, 66*(1), 104–117. doi:10 .1080/0312407X.2012.697566

Hinds, T., & Giardino, A. (2020). Compassion fatigue, burnout, and coping strategies among child-serving professionals. In *Child sexual abuse. Springer briefs in public health* (pp. 95–102). Springer. https://doi.org/10.1007/ 978-3-030-52549-1_4

Hunt, S., Goddard, C., Cooper, J., Littlechild, B., & Wild, J. (2016). 'If I feel like this, how does the child feel?' Child protection workers, supervision, management and organisational responses to parental violence. *Journal of Social Work Practice, 30*(1), 5–24. doi:10.1080/02650533.2015.10 73145

International Society for Traumatic Stress Studies. (2022, January 5). *Trauma basics.* https://istss.org/public-resources/trauma-basics

Jankoski, J. (2010). Is vicarious trauma the culprit? A study of child welfare professionals. *Child Welfare, 89*(6), 105–131.

Kaminski, M. (2001). Unintended consequences: Organizational practices and their impact on workplace safety and productivity. *Journal of Occupational Health Psychology, 6*(2), 127–138. doi:10.1037/1076-8998.6.2.127

Kezelman, C., & Stavropoulos, P. (2012). *The last frontier: Practice guidelines for treatment of complex trauma and trauma informed care and service delivery.* Adults Surviving Child Abuse.

King, M., Smith, A., & Gracey, M. (2009). Indigenous health part 2: The underlying causes of the health gap. *The Lancet, 374*(9683), 76–85. doi:10.1016/ S0140-6736(09)60827-8

Knight, C. (2015). Trauma informed social work practice: Practice considerations and challenges. *Clinical Social Work Journal, 43*(1), 25–37. doi:10.1007/ s10615-014-0481-6

Leblanc, V. R. (2009). The effects of acute stress on performance: Implications for health professions education. *Academic Medicine, 84*(10), S25–S33. doi:10.1097/ACM.0b013e3181b37b8f

Levy, M., & Poertner, J. (2014). Development of a child welfare worker stress inventory. *Journal of Psychological Issues in Organizational Culture, 5*(1), 7–15. doi:10.1002/jpoc.21134

Lewig, K., & McLean, S. (2016). *Caring for our frontline child protection workforce* (CFCA Paper No. 42). Child Family Community Australia Information Exchange, Australian Institute of Family Studies.

Littlechild, B. (2005). The nature and effects of violence against childprotection social workers: Providing effective support. *The British Journal of Social Work, 35*(3), 387–401. doi:10.1093/bjsw/bch188

Lowe, S., Okubo, Y., & Reilly, M. (2012). A qualitative inquiry into racism, trauma, and coping: Implications for supporting victims of racism. *Professional Psychology: Research and Practice, 43*(3), 190–198. doi:10.1037/a0026501

Menzies, K., & Gilbert, S. (2013). Engaging communities. In B. Bennett, S. Green, S. Gilbert, & D. Bessarab (Eds.), *Our voices: Aboriginal and Torres Strait Islander social work* (pp. 50–69). Palgrave Macmillan.

Meyer, E. C., Zimering, R., Daly, E., Knight, J., Kamholz, B. W., & Gulliver, S. B. (2012). Predictors of posttraumatic stress disorder and other psychological symptoms in trauma-exposed firefighters. *Psychological Services, 9*(1), 1–15. doi:10.1037/a0026414

McFadden, P. (2020). Two sides of one coin? Relationships build resilience or contribute to burnout in child protection social work: Shared perspectives from leavers and stayers in Northern Ireland. *International Social Work, 63*(2), 164–176. doi:10.1177/0020872818788393

McFadden, P., Campbell, A., & Taylor, B. (2015). Resilience and burnout in child protection social work: Individual and organisational themes from a systematic literature review. *The British Journal of Social Work, 45*(5), 1546–1563. doi:10.1093/bjsw/bct210

McFarlane, A., & Bryant, R. (2007). Post-traumatic stress disorder in occupational settings: Anticipating and managing the risk. *Occupational Medicine (Oxford), 57*, 404–410. doi:10.1093/occmed/kqm070

Munro, E. (2010). *The Munro review of child protection: Interim report – The child's journey.* Department of Education.

Oates, F. (2019). You are not allowed to tell: Organisational culture as a barrier for child protection workers seeking assistance for traumatic stress symptomology. *Children Australia, 44*(2), 84–90. doi:10.1017/cha.2019.12

Oates, F. (2020). Racism as trauma: Experiences of aboriginal and Torres Strait Islander Australian child protection practitioners. *Child Abuse & Neglect, 110*(Pt 3), 104262–104262. doi:10.1016/j.chiabu.2019.104262

Parks, K., & Steelman, L. (2008). Organizational wellness programs: A meta-analysis. *Journal of Occupational Health Psychology, 13*(1), 58–68. doi:10.1037/1076-8998.13.1.58

Pearlman, L. (1995). Self-care for trauma therapists: Ameliorating vicarious traumatization. In B. Stamm & A. Hudnall (Eds.), *Secondary traumatic stress: Self-care issues for clinicians, researchers, and educators* (pp. 51–64). The Sidran Press.

Pearlman, L., & Saakvitne, K. (1995). *Trauma and the therapist: Countertransference and vicarious traumatization in psychotherapy with incest survivors.* Norton.

Pyevich, C., Newman, E., & Daleiden, E (2003). The relationship among cognitive schemas, job-related traumatic exposure, and posttraumatic stress disorder in journalists. *Journal of Traumatic Stress, 16*(4), 325–328. doi:10.1023/A:1024405716529

Rantanen, M., Mauno, S., Kinnunen, U., & Rantanen, U. (2011). Do individual coping strategies help or harm in the work – family conflict situation? Examining coping as a moderator between work – family conflict and well-being. *International Journal of Stress Management, 18*(1), 24–48. doi:10.1037/a0022007

Regehr, C. (2018). *Stress, trauma, and decision-making for social workers.* Columbia University Press.

Rubino, C., Luksyte, A., Perry, S., & Volpone, S. (2009). How do stressors lead to burnout? The mediating role of motivation. *Journal of Occupational Health Psychology, 14*(3), 289–304. doi:10.1037/a0015284

Searle, B. (2008). Does personal initiative training work as a stress management intervention? *Journal of Occupational Health Psychology, 13*(3), 259–270. doi:10.1037/1076-8998.13.3.259

Sherwood, J. (2013). Colonisation – It's bad for your health: The context of Aboriginal health. *Contemporary Nurse, 46*(1), 28–40. doi:10.5172/conu.2013.46.1.28

Substance Abuse and Mental Health Services Administration. (2014). *SAMHSA's concept of trauma and guidance for a trauma informed approach.* Substance Abuse and Mental Health Services Administration.

Wall, L., Higgins, D., & Hunter, C. (2016). *Trauma informed care in child/family welfare services* (CFCA Paper No. 37). Child Family Community Australia information exchange, Australian Institute of Family Studies.

Whinghter, L. J., Cunningham, C. J. L., Wang, M., & Burnfield, J. L. (2008). The moderating role of goal orientation in the workload-frustration relationship. *Journal of Occupational Health Psychology, 13*(3), 283–291. doi:10.1037/1076-8998.13.3.283

Williams, A., Helm, H., & Clemens, E. (2012). The effect of childhood trauma, personal wellness, supervisory working alliance, and organizational factors on vicarious traumatization. *Journal of Mental Health Counseling, 34*(2), 133–153. doi:10.17744/mehc.34.2.j3l62k872325h583

Wise, S. (2017). *Developments to strengthen systems for child protection across Australia* (CFCA Paper No. 44). Child Family Community Australia Information Exchange, Australian Institute of Family Studies.

Zerubavel, N., & Wright, M. (2012). The dilemma of the wounded healer. *Psychotherapy, 49*(4), 482–491. doi:10.1037/a0027824

2 Supervision

What is supervision?

A large proportion of the literature pertaining to supervision that is relevant to those who work with vulnerable children and their families comes from the discipline of social work. The practice of supervision is deeply ingrained in the profession of social work and is taught widely in undergraduate social work degree programs. The definition of supervision relied on in the context of this book comes from social work academics Davys and Beddoe (2010), who cite that professional supervision is

> a forum for reflection and learning . . . an interactive dialogue between at least two people, one of whom is a supervisor. This dialogue shapes a process of review, reflection, critique and replenishment for professional practitioners. Supervision is a professional activity in which practitioners are engaged throughout the duration of their careers regardless of experience or qualification. The participants are accountable to professional standards and defined competencies and to organisational policy and procedures.
>
> (p. 21)

The definition outlined by academics Davys and Beddoe (2010) is also the definition relied on by the Australian Association of Social Workers (AASW, 2014). Other national social work associations include elements like accountability, ethical practice, lifelong learning, professional development, and critical reflection to be central in any model of effective supervision (BASW, 2011; ANZASW, 2016; CASW, 2020; NASW & ASWB, 2013). Although the definition relied on in this book comes from the discipline of social work, that does not exclude those

DOI: 10.4324/9781003026006-3

practitioners working in this field who have different training and/or qualifications. As we will discuss throughout this book, the concepts of supervision in a child welfare context are applicable across disciplines and practice settings.

In relation to supervision, Kadushin and Harkness (2014) write that there are three key elements to the functionality of supervision: administrative, educational and supportive. While there is wide acceptance of these three core elements of supervision in the literature (Beddoe & Davys, 2016; Berger & Quiros, 2016; Tsui, 2005), Rankine (2019) argues that a fourth key function, mediation, is also central. These four elements of supervision in combination are central to effective supervision practice. I will now discuss each of the four in some more detail.

The administrative element of supervision discussed in the literature pertains to matters that are organisationally driven. The purpose of administrative supervision is for the line supervisor or manager to ensure the practitioner is delivering services in an effective and efficient way that is consistent with organisational requirements. The administrative element in supervision is likely to include completion targets like number of home visits or case plans completed in a month, human resources requirements such as timesheets, leave planning or mandatory training requirements like fire safety and the storage of chemicals in the workplace. Administrative supervision facilitates the supervisor or manager's ability to manage their staff, manage the workload and flow of their work units and make clear to the practitioner what the organisational expectations of them are.

Managerial requirements often drive the necessity to focus on the administrative element of supervision. Political influence may also heavily affect levels of administrative supervision. As an example, if there had been a high-profile death of an infant resulting in negative media attention and public scrutiny, supervisors may be directed by senior executives in the organisation or perhaps a government minister's office to review all related open cases in newborn children. With a heavy focus on a particular age group, families with children outside of that age group may have less organisational attention. The literature is critical of these managerial and political drivers of supervision as this is often a factor in the focus on practitioner wellbeing and development being diverted (Hunt et al., 2016; Goddard & Hunt, 2011). There is, however, some praise in the literature for an increased focus on administration, as it is seen as a mechanism to embed accountability both in relation to public resources and service users (Nickson et al., 2019; Regehr, 2018).

The educational element of supervision discussed in the literature pertains to professional development activities encompassing both formal and informal learning opportunities. Brittain (2009) argues that the core purpose of the educational element in supervision is to furnish the practitioners with the skills, knowledge, experiences and attitudes required to successfully undertake their duties. Formal opportunities for the learning and integration of knowledge into practice may be a request for funds for a practitioner to attend specialist training or to subscribe to a professional peer-reviewed journal as a strategy to keep practitioner knowledge current. Informal opportunities may be engaging in live supervision, where a practitioner accompanies a more experienced practitioner, possibly the line supervisor, on home visits or to meetings where they can observe the application of professional knowledge into practice with clients and other stakeholders. A critically reflective session after such an opportunity presents a real and tangible space for a practitioner to solidify their knowledge base and increase their professional capacity to undertake their role successfully. These opportunities are consistent with the educational element of supervision in practice literature (Kadushin & Harkness, 2014).

The support element of supervision discussed in the literature pertains to both practitioner wellbeing matters and support to practitioners to achieve job satisfaction. Brittain's (2009) interpretation of the inclusion of job satisfaction as an optimal outcome of the supportive element of supervision is that increased job satisfaction among practitioners leads to increased motivation, good morale individually and within teams and sustained commitment to the organisation, leading to better outcomes for vulnerable clients. The things likely to be linked with the supportive element of traditional supervision might be the canvassing of self-care activities including the reduction of stress, active listening by the supervisor coupled with recognition of achievements and professional growth, acknowledgement of the difficulty undertaking such work, reassurance and encouragement. The support element of supervision is also highlighted in the literature as critical to assisting practitioners to manage the impact of vicarious and secondary trauma as well as other work-related stressors (Hunt et al., 2016; Kadushin & Harkness, 2014). Cole et al., (2006) and Ingram (2013) both support the notion that supervision that embraces and openly explores practitioner feeling of emotion in their practice with vulnerable people contributes positively to practitioner performance. Additionally, Tsang (2006) supports the need for supervision to have a replenishing and emotionally nourishing function. There is opposition to this in the literature which will be explored later in the book.

Deviating from the traditional three pillars of supervision is Morrison's (2001) inclusion of mediation as a fourth pillar. Morrison (2001) describes the mediation element of supervision to support a balance between practice knowledge and development, including wellbeing support, as well as the exploration of tensions that exist between the practitioner and the organisation. This element speaks to the ongoing negotiation in supervision between the needs and agenda of the practitioner and the needs and agenda of the organisation. Often these needs are in opposition to each other, creating a potential source of conflict within the supervision process.

Balancing the elements

Balancing the elements of supervision to meet both the needs of the organisation and those of the practitioner can be an ongoing struggle. There are many facets of supervision, all of which need to align, supported by the right resources, for the most effective outcome for all concerned. In a broader sense, this includes service users as well. The inclusion of mediation as an additional element to the traditional three of administrative, educational and supportive is a useful tool to assist with balance. Balancing of the three core elements of supervision to maximise effectiveness is supported in the supervision research literature (Davys & Beddoe, 2010; Kadushin & Harkness, 2014; Rankine, 2019). The mediation element of supervision supports a negotiation between service users, practitioners, managers, organisations and public expectations. Balance requires ongoing and deliberate maintenance, all of which takes time. Time in the child protection workplace is at a premium and a finite resource. A lack of time has been identified in the research literature to be a key factor in the poor delivery of supervision by both practitioners and supervisors (Hunt et al., 2016; McCrae et al., 2015; Oates, 2019).

It can be difficult for the practitioner to balance the elements of supervision. Supervision is a forum where practitioners should feel supported to discuss matters pertaining to their wellbeing. However, due to organisational operational need, sessions can tend to focus on the management of client-related tasks and the management of workloads. The administrative element of supervision is often prioritised over the support and educational element of supervision. The prioritising of the administrative element of supervision at the expense of the supportive and educational elements can be problematic for the practitioner over the medium to long term. The lack of focus on the supportive element may leave practitioners vulnerable to occupational trauma, impeding their ability to undertake their work with vulnerable children and families. Similarly, the educational element of supervision furnishes a practitioner with the skills and knowledge to successfully undertake their work. A lack of focus on this element may contribute to gaps in practitioner knowledge or the ability to translate research, theories or frameworks into frontline practice with vulnerable children and families. O'Donoghue (2015) argues that supervision should be separated into portfolios as a strategy to manage the elements of supervision more effectively. Research literature supports the separation of some elements of traditional line supervision (like the managerial aspects) from the support element of supervision (Hunt et al., 2016; O'Donoghue, 2015; Rankine, 2019) as a way of ensuring practitioners receive all elements equally. The delicate balance for supervisors and managers between managing organisational expectations around workload and acknowledging and managing practitioners who may be exhibit symptoms of occupational stress will be discussed in more detail later.

Supervision in a child welfare occupational context

As discussed, supervision in a child welfare practice context is identified in the literature as a process facilitated by an experienced practitioner, often a worker's line supervisor, that has an educational, supportive and administrative focus (Berger & Quiros, 2016; Davys & Beddoe, 2010) as well as a mediation element (Rankine, 2019). I also previously discussed the consensus in the literature that good supervision is a significant contributing factor to supporting practitioners by reducing the effect of occupational trauma and other trauma-related illness, as well as strengthening practitioner satisfaction in their work and retention in their role (Gibbs, 2001; Hunt et al., 2016; Manthorpe et al., 2015). Professional supervision can be delivered in a range of modes and mediums. The most commonly used type of supervision in a child welfare practice setting is internal or external supervision or a combination of both. I will spend some time exploring both internal and external supervision, what they are, their purpose, benefits and challenges.

Internal supervision

Internal supervision is the most common type of supervision offered to practitioners who work with vulnerable children and their families.

Internal supervision occurs in the workplace in a one-on-one inter-action between a practitioner and usually their line supervisor or manager. Frequency and expectation to attend varies widely between organisations and at times between disciplines. Egan's (2012) study of Australian social workers found that two-thirds received internal supervision only, with the balance receiving a combination of supervision opportunities to supplement their internal supervision.

There is criticism in the literature about the quality of internal supervision offered to child protection practitioners particularly those working in statutory contexts. Studies by Manthorpe et al. (2015); Wilkins et al., (2017); and Goddard and Hunt (2011) all found that the provision of supervision to practitioners working with vulner-able children and families was heavily weighted towards compliance, driven by organisational agendas and lacked a clear focus on reflec-tive practice and practitioner wellbeing.

In my own research pertaining to supervision in the child protec-tion workplace, I found that the experience of practitioners working in a non-statutory context to be markedly different to those working in a statutory child protection context. Practitioners working in non-statutory environments described internal supervision to be very use-ful both in managing both their workloads and their wellbeing.

> *It is fantastic . . . community sector are much better at it, much better at supporting workers. (Matilda)*
> *It's very good. (Missy)*
> *It's been really good. (Grace)*

However, practitioners with statutory child protection work experi-ence largely reported poor access to internal supervision, which they described to be administrative, task focused, compliance based, incon-sistent and often not meeting their professional or practice needs:

> *It is very, very tasky. (Isabella)*
> *My idea of supervision coming from social work was very different to what I found when I came to [government department] because the idea of supervision in [government department] was, 'Let's look at your board. Let's look at what cases you've got. Let's talk through that', and that usu-ally takes an hour. 'Have you got any leave coming up?' 'No.' 'Alright, fine. You may leave now'. Whereas social work supervision is more critical reflection: How can I improve my practice? How can I link my theoreti-cal understanding of social work practice to what I'm actually doing on the ground? How can I engage with some self-care practices? That was*

my idea of supervision and so at first I was a little disappointed by the supervision that was available in [government department]. The only way I could solve that was by seeking external supervision with the social worker outside of [government department]. (Alice)

Many practitioners outlined that the internal supervision available to them in their statutory child protection workplace did not tend to focus on their wellbeing or self-care needs:

> *I think it's good to have supervision with your [line supervisor]. I think that's required, I think that's needed. I think cases need to be discussed. But on the other hand, [practitioners] need to have that emotional debriefing about how it's impacting on them along the way . . . supervision [at statutory agency] was more about getting the job done, paperwork-based type thing, compared to worrying about how I felt or what I was going through at the time. It was very bang, bang, bang, get the job done, bang, bang, bang, get the paperwork done. 'You should have this, this and this done by now. Why haven't you?' (Rosalyn)*
>
> *It certainly wasn't about my wellbeing and it was generally me organising it. But definitely not about me, that's why I burnt out, because I had no support. (Matilda)*

External supervision

The second most common mode of supervision undertaken by professionals working with vulnerable children and their families is external supervision. External supervision in a child welfare occupational context usually refers to the provision of supervision to practitioners by a more experienced practitioner outside of their organisation. These sessions can be funded either by a practitioner's organisation or by the practitioner themselves. Some organisations offer a combination, where the practitioner might fund sessions themselves with their organisation allowing attendance during paid work time. In some jurisdictions, the cost of external supervision sessions can be claimed as a work-related expense for taxation purposes, allowing practitioners to claim the cost back at a later time. Some practitioners will choose to undertake external supervision with a practitioner of the same professional or qualification background like psychology or nursing. This can be related to satisfying professional association requirements to maintain currency, especially for professionals working in multidisciplinary teams where line supervisors may not have the same professional background as those they supervise.

In my own research, almost all participants stated their preference for external supervision over the internal models of supervision that would usually be delivered by their line supervisors in their place of work. A key difference between practitioner experiences of internal and external supervision was that they felt that external supervision was a safe place to explore issues pertaining to their wellbeing whereas internal supervision was more about 'cases', organisational compliance and other administrative tasks. Speaking specifically about the difficulties experienced being constantly exposed to trauma as part of their role, many practitioners viewed external supervision to be an essential strategy for managing their wellbeing:

> *I think it needs to happen everywhere, and particularly in somewhere like child protection because I think that – the issue is, is that people kind of lose themselves in that organisation because they just become so entrenched in the trauma and the, you know, the heartache that goes on. Their hearts either become super hard, or they break. (Matilda)*
>
> *You're able to go and get things off your chest. The weight off your shoulder. For your own mental wellbeing, because what we take on every day is huge. To be able to talk to people and get stuff off your chest on hard cases is important. (Missy)*
>
> *I think that outside supervision is good just to have that, you know, if stuff's building up and you're not able to talk to anybody, then you've got somebody that you can actually go out and talk to and it's somebody that you've chosen yourself. (Lisa)*

Many practitioners shared that external supervision offered them a place of safety where they could discuss matters, both personal and work related, without fear. Participants used words such as 'freedom', 'safe' and 'private' to describe their experiences with external supervision. The participants expressed a reluctance to articulate their needs fully during internal supervision primarily because of fear of being judged unfairly by their supervisor or being viewed as incompetent:

> *You risk judgement being passed from a supervisor. So it's more about just sharing what you need to share within a work framework. Whereas the external one is unloading without the fear of 'my boss is going to take this and do something with it', or 'and it's going to go on my file'. It is somewhere safe to go. (David)*
>
> *It just gave me the freedom, I suppose, to feel like, okay, whoever I'm talking to, it's definitely not – there's no connection to [participant's workplace] in any way. (Alice)*

*I can tell [external supervisor] anything and everything and she lis-
tens and advises me. But yeah, she doesn't have that connection back here.
Because I feel you just don't – when you work in a place where you're not
fully trusting of everyone within that organisation, it can be a concern
if you want to go yarn to someone about something. So the fact that you
can go and talk to someone totally outside of [participant's workplace] is
good. Very good. (Missy)*

Participant Alice reported experiencing substantial benefits from
external supervision, particularly in relation to her wellbeing:

*I don't think I would have lasted with [government department] or in
child protection. I probably would have started to be one of those jaded
people that thought child protection was a horrible place. (Alice)*

While the participants in my research only reported positive experiences with external supervision, they did discuss a number of issues
related to access. Two main access issues emerged from analysis of
the participants' narratives: cost and time. The cost of contracting an
external supervisor without the financial support of the workplace,
at least in part, was described as a factor that would restrict access to
external supervision for many practitioners:

*You know, $150 or $160 a month for a session is sometimes out of our
reach . . . they give you the time off, but you have to actually pay for it.
(Elvina)*
*   I think if the [government agency] was to say, 'We will give you this
money for some external supervision', then I think more people would take
it up. I would like to advocate for [government department] to fund that
for their staff because I think it puts a lot of pressure on if you're expected
to fund it yourself. (Alice)*

Others described the issue of time as a critical factor pertaining
to accessing external supervision. The participants stated that,
because of their heavy workloads, even if the workplace approved
time for external supervision, they felt they would be unable to
access it. Many stated that they would need to access external supervision during worktime because of heavy family commitments after
hours:

*I'm happy to cover the cost, but I need to do it during work time. So I've
written that into my plan. (Isabella)*

I mean, I had asked for it at [government department], but, yeah, it was 'pay for it yourself, do it in your own time'. (Matilda)

As mentioned, the child protection practitioners in my own research categorically agreed that external supervision was their preferred model of supervision, particularly in relation to managing matters pertaining to wellbeing, practice and professional development.

Considerations for First Nations practitioners

In an Australian context, there has been much debate about the role of cultural supervision and the benefits to Aboriginal and/or Torres Strait Islander child protection practitioners. The provision of cultural supervision to First Nations practitioners has also been widely discussed in such countries as Canada and New Zealand. In my own research I asked practitioners about their views on cultural supervision and their thoughts on Indigenous Australian practitioners having access to an Indigenous supervisor. In relation to the cultural background of the professional supervisor, that is, whether or not they themselves identified as Aboriginal or Torres Strait Islander, there was no consensus among the practitioners. Some stated they did not have a preference for an Indigenous or non-Indigenous supervisor:

Well, it's like my supervisor coming into that system supervising me, whether it's Black or white or whatever origin. The supervisor just needs to have those skills. (Elvina)

Others stated that they would prefer an Indigenous supervisor; however, if one was unavailable, then a non-Indigenous supervisor would be suitable:

I had a couple of people at work that I could talk to – that was good enough for me. But I think if an Indigenous person had an Indigenous person to speak to, they would have better understanding of the historical stuff and be able to identify and relate to some of the issues that that person was going through at the time. (Rosalyn)

One participant stated that having access to an Indigenous supervisor was a non-negotiable for them:

There's just something about our shared experience and our shared inherent histories that connects us more than what it would to a white person.

So, like, if you talk about Stolen Generation, she's going to have her story, I'll have my story. That's what connects us. Whereas it's not going to be the case for white people. (Isabella)

The varied views of practitioners in the study indicated that Indigenous Australian child protection practitioners do not have homogenous supervision and support needs. Matilda stated:

We're all individuals. You know, like, you can't say all Aboriginal people are the same, and all Torres Strait Islanders are the same. We all come from different backgrounds, you know, it's not just about the culture itself, it's about all of those other cultural things, like, you know, what family means to us – we are part of a group, another sort of group. To me, I think that it's more about – I think it's more about having information and having support available to all staff when it comes to cultural matters. (Matilda)

Matilda's view that Indigenous practitioners do not have homogenous supervision and support needs is consistent with Berlin (2002), who argued that:

classifying people on the basis of group membership only gives us the illusion that we are being culturally sensitive, when, in fact, we are failing to look beyond easy characterisations for the particular and specific ways that *this* person is understanding, feeling and acting.

(p. 144)

The narratives of those who participated in my own research provide further evidence that supervision and support needs are unique to individual practitioners and that a 'one size fits all' approach will not provide adequately for the needs of practitioners.

The use of supervision across non-traditional practice settings

The chapter thus far has explored supervision, its purpose and place within a child protection workplace context. Most services, either government administered or government funded programs aimed at working with vulnerable children and their families, have mandatory or internal policies and procedures about the timely provision of professional supervision for professional staff. However, this practice context is not the only setting where such work is under-taken. In the Introduction to this book I outlined some of the practice settings where practitioners who undertake child welfare work are not considered traditional providers of such work, like nurses, doctors, law and justice professionals, professionals working in schools and other education settings. These practice settings are often defined under different service delivery banners, like universal health care, education or services pertaining to the justice system; however, they are critical parts of the child protection continuum. It is professionals working in non-traditional child welfare settings who, in my view, are often overlooked in the discussion about access to quality and responsive supervision. As an example, nurses across jurisdictions are often the professionals who first come into contact with children who have experienced significant abuse and/or neglect. These practice settings may be through hospitals where children may present with significant injuries or through child and maternal health care services. While nurses are more likely to have contact with children and families where child protection concerns may be present, they are less likely to have access to supervision. As an example, although recommended by peak bodies, it is not a requirement for nurses to receive clinical supervision (Driscoll et al., 2019).

Educational professionals are also likely to be the first professionals in a child's life to detect a child's experience of child abuse and/or neglect. However, there are studies (Hunt & Broadley, 2020; Tillman et al., 2016), that indicate strong reticence by educational professionals to report suspected child abuse and neglect to child protection authorities. Key reasons for non-reporting of suspected child abuse included a lack of education of what constitutes child abuse and neglect, what evidence is required when making a report and also difficulties managing conflicting emotions like the desire not to break up families unnecessarily. These barriers could all be addressed by the provision of responsive supervision, underpinned by the four core elements of quality supervision outlined previously in this chapter: administrative, educational, supportive and mediation.

Barriers to receiving effective supervision in child protection

As previously mentioned, the research literature is clear that the provision of quality responsive supervision to professionals working in trauma-laden environments is critical to their overall wellbeing and capacity to undertake their duties. What is also clear in the research literature is the continued struggle organisations have that deliver services to vulnerable children and their families when it comes to providing supervision and other forms of support to their staff. Barriers for organisations responsively supporting staff working in trauma-laden environments will be explored in more detail in the coming chapter; however, I will briefly touch on it now for context. In the research literature regarding difficulty providing supervision to professionals working with vulnerable children and their families, two key themes are identified repeatedly. These barriers are organisational, specifically organisational culture and organisational resourcing, and practitioner perception.

Organisational culture

Organisational culture is identified strongly in the literature as being a key barrier to practitioners accessing support and supervision, especially in a child welfare context. With mounting political pressure, increasing public suspicion of welfare services, negative media attention and the ever-looming threat of budget cuts, the pressure not to make mistakes has never been greater. The increasingly risk-averse nature of child protection work has created great apprehension in the administrative levels of organisations, resulting in strong reluctance to think outside the box or to try new things in preference for organisational compliance.

The risk-averse nature of practice with vulnerable children and their families contributes to the lack of support available for practitioners through internal supervision. Organisational and political priorities often necessitate a line supervisor's focus in supervision on procedural compliance in case work. While of course the goal of any supervisor is to ensure quality evidence-based services are delivered to clients, the shift in focus is organisationally driven, often by executive administrators, and is therefore often beyond the control of individual supervisors and line managers.

Also included under the theme of organisational culture as a barrier is the hesitancy for practitioners who may be experiencing occupational traumatic stress to seek support from line supervisors, managers and even peers for fear of a negative outcome. In my own research (Oates, 2019), practitioners expressed their strong reluctance to voice their experiences of occupational traumatic stress for fear of being ridiculed or ostracised, labelled as incompetent, not 'cut out' for child protection work or sanctioned as retribution for speaking out.

Practitioners also identified concern that their career prospects, like promotions, could be negatively affected.

Organisational resourcing

Organisational resourcing, or more aptly lack of resourcing, is another key barrier identified in the research literature to organisations providing practitioners with access to supervision. The rise of managerialism in social welfare has restricted the ability of organisations to provide optimal levels of support to staff. Increasing cuts to public funding for social service provision has resulted in tighter budget considerations for government and non-government services. In times of cost cutting and austerity measures, staff supervision and training costs are often the first to be limited. While a number of organisations support individual practitioners to access external supervision, some during paid work time, practitioners frequently cite cost as a barrier that negatively affects their ability to participate without the financial support of their employer. Even if practitioners do find themselves able to access external or other supplementary supervision supports through their organisation, increasing case complexity and numbers of clients limit their ability to access supervision during paid work hours. Accessing external supports outside of paid work hours is an option offered to practitioners in a number of organisations. However, the viability of this option is precarious for the predominantly female workforce who often have caring responsibilities that preclude them from attending after-hours engagements.

Practitioner perception

Practitioner perception of what supervision is, what the sessions will be used for and what the benefit is for them is frequently cited in the research literature as a barrier to practitioner engagement. Practitioner suspicion that supervision, internal supervision in particular, is a method of organisational surveillance or a quasi performance management exercise has been frequently reported (Beddoe & Davys, 2016; Gilbert, 2001). Johns (2001) is critical of internal models of supervision, stating that 'supervision . . . becomes an opportunity to shape the practitioner into organisationally preferred ways of practice, even whilst veiled as being in the practitioner's best interests' (p. 140). The literature supports the criticism by practitioners that internal supervision is more often than not an exercise in organisational compliance rather than a safe professional space to critically reflect on oneself and the work being undertaken with vulnerable children and their families (Bradbury-Jones, 2013; Hunt et al., 2016). With practitioners managing multiple competing and often urgent priorities, practitioners see attending supervision sessions as not an optimal use of their time.

The supervisor and the supervisory relationship

One of the key elements of effective supervision is of course the supervisor – specifically, the supervisory relationship. The research literature is clear that the supervisory relationship is a critical factor in the successful experience of supervision by practitioners. As an example, a study by Beddoe et al. (2014), found that regularity of supervision was not enough to effectively support practitioners. The supervisory relationship in combination with regularity was central. Strong, professional relationships between a supervisor and practitioner have been found to contribute positively towards a practitioner's ability to move through occupational stress (Beddoe et al., 2014; Berger & Quiros, 2016; McPherson et al., 2016), critically explore and improve practice (Little et al., 2018; Radey & Stanley, 2018), build professional resiliency (Beddoe et al., 2014; Regehr, 2018) and increase rates of job satisfaction (Hunt et al., 2016; Regehr, 2018).

In addition to the supervisor's ability to build trust and safety within the supervisory relationship, the research literature indicated consensus on other key elements that lead to the creation and maintenance of a successful supervisory relationship as defined by supervisees. These attributes included availability, consistency and predictability (Berger & Quiros, 2016; McPherson et al., 2016; Radey & Stanley, 2018); acknowledgement of own limitations and humility (Berger & Quiros, 2016); fostering a learning and professional development culture (Berger & Quiros, 2016; Little et al., 2018); valued staff (McPherson et al., 2016); experienced and knowledgeable (Kouzes & Posner, 2016; Rankine, 2019); empathetic, self-regulating and encouraging of self-care (Abassary & Goodrich, 2014; McPherson et al., 2016; Radey & Stanley, 2018).

In my own research, practitioners outlined a number of attributes that they felt contributed positively to their experience of supervision while they were undertaking their role working with children and families where child protection concerns were present. One stand-out attribute was the work history of the supervisor. There was consensus among the practitioners that an effective supervisor had to have a professional background of working in child protection.

You do need a likeminded person to debrief with. (Elvina)

Yeah, just so that they can understand what it is that you're actually talking about and why you're perhaps feeling that way. (David)

I have two people that I go between because they give me different needs and both of them, particularly, have worked in the Indigenous space, as in with children and families, workers, organisations. So those two are the only ones that I'll go to. I won't go to anybody else. (Isabella)

Practitioners felt that speaking with a supervisor who has previously worked in the area of child protection afforded them a level of comfort and freedom in their sessions:

I tend to use humour as a defence mechanism, but because of my work in child protection, I have a very dark sense of humour. So I would tell jokes during our sessions and if I had told that joke to somebody who didn't have that background, I think it would have been more uncomfortable, whereas for her, she got the joke, she got the fact that I needed to use my sense of humour in that way. Yeah, so that was also good. That was very liberating. (Alice)

Because she's got a strong child protection background, she's able to give me some good advice as well. If it was just a psychologist that was general and didn't know the child protection stuff, I think I'd just be trying to explain myself a bit more. Whereas I can just straight off the bat yarn to her about a case and she knows exactly the processes and exactly what should have happened or should be happening and will advise me on what to do. (Missy)

Threats to a successful supervisory relationship

While the supervisory relationship can contribute to a practitioner's personal and professional growth, it can also be the source of great angst and difficulty for both the practitioner and the supervisor. Consistent with the research literature, practitioners in my own research identified supervisor commitment to supervision as a critical element for the building and maintenance of a successful supervisory relationship. A lack of commitment, perceived or otherwise, by supervisors was a key element identified by practitioners as a threat to a successful supervisory relationship. Cancelled or perpetually postponed supervision sessions due to the emergence of 'more important' matters were commonly experienced:

> *I think the biggest thing is inconsistency and that's why I ended up finding the issue is, yeah, we have one month and then we reschedule for the next one because we were either both busy or our schedules didn't allow for a supervision session because something pops up. So you've got to go and deal with that. So it needs to be set in stone, it needs to be regular, it needs to be consistent.* (David)

Some participants stated that regular formal supervision was never scheduled in their statutory workplace:

> *I could probably count on my two hands the number of times I had supervision in that [number] years.* (Matilda)
> *I wasn't a statutory officer. I didn't require supervision [supervision not mandatory], but even the statutory officers didn't get supervision.* (Sarah)

Some participants described asking for supervision and their request not being fulfilled, or, in some cases, being scolded by their line supervisor for asking:

> *She came back and she went, 'I'm not your mother. I don't need to hold your hand and sit down and talk to you and rub your back for an hour every week. If you've got a problem, come and see me. I have an open door and you are not children'.* (Mary)

A functional supervisory relationship is a key element underpinning good quality and responsive support to practitioners working in trauma-laden environments. Exploration of this dynamic from the supervisory and organisational point of view inclusive of case studies will continue in subsequent chapters.

Trauma informed supervision

As outlined previously, supervision is generally a reflective exercise undertaken by practitioners with a more experienced colleague, usually their line supervisor. It is an opportunity to explore practice challenges, unpack ethical dilemmas, discuss workloads, and tend to wellbeing matters. It is clear that the provision of good quality supervision that is not solely administrative or driven by organisational agendas is hugely beneficial both to the practitioner and the vulnerable clients they provide services to.

The concept of trauma informed practice is now ubiquitous is the social service delivery landscape in relation to working with vulnerable people. However, trauma informed ways of working with practitioners are patchy at best. In the previous chapter, I introduced six principles that were agreed on in the literature to be the foundation of a trauma informed approach. Those six principles are safety; trustworthiness and transparency; peer support; collaboration and mutuality; empowerment, voice and choice; and cultural, historical and gender considerations (SAMHSA, 2014). I will now discuss each of these six principles and how they can form the framework of trauma informed supervision with professionals who work with vulnerable children and their families.

Safety: The safety principle refers to both the physical and psychological safety of staff in a work group or organisation. Safety in this context can be the perceived sense of safety rather than the actuality of safety. As an example, undertaking front-line roles where the assessment of parental risks to children is inherently dangerous. Therefore, exposure to violence is an occupational hazard, the risk of which cannot always be mitigated. Safety in this instance would relate to the practitioner's belief that their work environment, including their peers and managers, would care for them in a genuine, supportive and responsive way should either their physical or psychological safety be threatened or breached. The feeling that colleagues and managers would support a practitioner when their safety threshold has been breached would also extend to professional safety in a child welfare context. An example of this may be when practitioners find themselves the subject of inquiries or investigations in relation to assessments they've made. While these inquiries are common in a child welfare context when a child has been injured or killed by a parent or when a parent or community member has made a complaint about a practitioner, the investigation process can be isolating, with many practitioners reported to feel scapegoated by their organisation.

Trustworthiness and transparency: This principle in a staff context relates to a sense of shared trust between a practitioner and the organisation that employs them. The goal attached to this principle is for trust to be built and maintained that is mutual between practitioners and their employing organisations. This could be achieved by transparent and consultative decision making around operations of a workplace. Examples could include the way staff leave is taken, processes around recording staff whereabouts, how workloads are distributed or what kind of professional development funds and activities are allocated and when. Similar to the safety principle, the perception of trust and transparency for the practitioner can be as important as actual transparency or where transparency cannot be achieved. An example of this might be if a decision is mandated by a statutory authority or where sensitive matters preclude all staff from knowing particular details and therefore collaborative decision making would be inappropriate.

Peer support: The peer support principle relates to support accessed by a practitioner from peers who share similar experiences. That could mean others who do the same job, work in the same field or have experienced the same event. It is a shared understanding amongst peers where mutual or reciprocal support is the goal. In the child welfare organisational context, it is important for supervisors and line managers to support, value and even actively encourage practitioners to engage in peer support processes in the business as usual context as well as in times of crisis. Without organisational endorsement, formal or otherwise, practitioners may be reluctant to openly engage in such endeavours, especially during work time, for fear of being viewed as non-productive or disruptive.

Collaboration and mutuality: The collaboration and mutuality principle places partnership as central. Healing is viewed as a collaborative undertaking involving practitioners and clients as well as the organisation, as appropriate. All the actors within this healing framework are viewed as having an important role. Identification and analysis of power constructs are a key component to facilitating genuine collaborative processes. What this may look like in a workplace setting is the use of 360-degree feedback, satisfaction surveys that are valued and the outcomes implemented. Implementation could be the use of the feedback to review and evaluate program delivery or to inform new service delivery offerings. Another example may be the creation of a reference group that genuinely values and integrates the views of people with lived experience.

Empowerment, voice and choice: The empowerment, voice and choice element of a trauma informed framework supports clients to genuinely participate in goal setting and decision making about their lives. Lived experiences of both the client and the practitioner are acknowledged, valued and seen as strengths to be built upon. The tenets of recovery and healing underpin the work of the practitioner with clients and the operations of the organisation.

Cultural, historical and gender considerations: The cultural, historical and gender considerations element acknowledges the oppression and lived experience of marginalised groups like women, First Nations peoples, those living with disability and members of LGBTIQA+ communities as examples. The organisational support needs of practitioners as well as clients from these groups are identified and policies and procedures designed and implemented in collaboration to ensure further oppression and marginalisation does not occur. Practitioners and organisations will actively seek and be open to the views of these groups and be prepared to effect changes.

When reviewing the six elements as a whole, there are a few themes that are common to most of the elements. One key theme is the acknowledgement of practitioners' lived experience of trauma. Another is the identification, analysis and challenging of power constructs within all aspects of service delivery and organisational operations inclusive of practitioners and clients.

Working with practitioners who have a history of trauma

Whilst the research literature is patchy when it comes to the number of practitioners who enter this field of work with a lived experience of trauma, anecdotally the percentage is high. It is often the case that this field of work draws those who have experienced similar circumstances to the client group being serviced or have loved ones who have. Safety and empowerment creation within the supervisory relationship is a critical element for practitioners to feel able to deconstruct their own histories of trauma and to safely and critically reflect on the possible connection to emerging occupational trauma symptomology. Authors like Berger and Quiros (2016), Harris and Fallot (2001) and McPherson et al. (2016) have argued that a supervisee's feeling of safety and a supervisor's ability to create it are essential elements required for an effective trauma informed supervisory relationship. The ability of supervisors to facilitate a practitioner's sharing of emotional distress and to safely lead them to a place where critical reflection and eventually integrated learning can occur is critical to the professional development of the practitioner as well as a strategy to safeguard against internalising occupational traumatic stress.

Authors such as Berger and Quiros (2016) and Jankoski (2010) concur that organisations must invest in regular and consistent trauma informed supervision for their employees. It is my view that organisations that work with traumatised populations would benefit from psycho-education regarding the experience of occupational trauma, including how symptoms manifest in the workplace. This psycho-education should also extend to practitioners. Increased awareness will increase a practitioner's ability to identify symptomology of occupational traumatic stress within themselves which indicates they may need to seek out additional supports.

Chapter summary

In this chapter we have explored the concept and purpose of supervision generally as well as in a child welfare organisational context. The supervisory relationship has been explored, focusing on what elements are present in strong supervisory relationships and what elements may constitute a threat. Trauma informed supervision was introduced as a concept, including how elements of a trauma informed approach to supervision may assist practitioners to work through occupational traumatic stress as well as issues that may arise due to their own lived experience of trauma while undertaking their paid duties. In the next chapter, the impact of managerialism on the core business of organisations and their ability to provide quality supervision that is responsive to the professional and wellbeing needs of practitioners will be discussed. Also included are case studies that have been drawn from the human and social services field that outline challenges and dilemmas faced by supervisors and managers.

Reflective questions for practice

1. As a practitioner working in a trauma-laden environment, what would your support and supervision needs be?
2. What specifically would be beneficial for your supervisor to be aware of to strengthen their ability to support your professional and wellbeing needs?

References

Abassary, C., & Goodrich, K. (2014). Attending to crisis-based supervision for counselors: The CARE model of crisis-based supervision. *The Clinical Supervisor, 33*(1), 63–81. doi:10.1080/07325223.2014.918006

Aotearoa New Zealand Association of Social Workers. (2016). *ANZASW supervision policy.* https://anzasw.nz/wp-content/uploads/ANZASW-Supervision-Policy-Updated-August-2016.pdf

Australian Association of Social Workers. (2014). *Supervision standards.* AASW.

Beddoe, L., & Davys, A. (2016). *Challenges in professional supervision: Current themes and models for practice.* Jessica Kingsley Publishers.

Beddoe, L., Davys, A., & Adamson, C. (2014). Never trust anybody who says 'I don't need supervision': Practitioners' beliefs about social worker resilience. *Practice* (Birmingham, England), *26*(2), 113–130. https://doi.org/1 0.1080/09503153.2014.896888

Berger, R., & Quiros, L. (2016). Best practices for training trauma informed practitioners: Supervisors' voice. *Traumatology, 22*(2), 145–154. doi:10.1037/ trm0000076

Berlin, S. (2002). *Clinical social work practice: A cognitive-integrative perspective.* Oxford University Press.

Bradbury-Jones, C. (2013). Refocusing child protection supervision: An innovative approach to supporting practitioners. *Child Care in Practice, 19*(3), 253–266. doi:10.1080/13575279.2013.785937

British Association of Social Workers. (2011). *UK supervision policy.* British Association of Social Workers.

Brittain, C. (2009). Models of social work supervision. In C. Potter & C. Brittain (Eds.), *Child welfare supervision: A practical guide for supervisors, managers and administrators* (pp. 23–43). Oxford University Press.

Canadian Association of Social Workers. (2020). *Scope of practice statement.* www. casw-acts.ca/files/attachements/Scope_of_Practice_Statement_2020_1.pdf

Cole, M., Bruch, H., & Vogel, B. (2006). Emotion as mediators of the relations between perceived supervisor support and psychological hardiness on employee cynicism. *Journal of Organizational Behavior, 27*(4), 463–484. https://doi.org/10.1002/job.381

Davys, A., & Beddoe, L. (2010). *Best practice in professional supervision: A guide for the helping professions.* Jessica Kingsley.

Driscoll, J., Stacey, G., Harrison-Dening, K., Boyd, C., & Shaw, T. (2019). Enhancing the quality of clinical supervision in nursing practice. *Nursing Standard, 34*(5), 43–50. https://doi.org/10.7748/ns.2019.e11228

Egan, R. (2012). Australian social work supervision practice in 2007. *Australian Social Work, 65*(2), 171–184. https://doi.org/10.1080/0312407X. 2011.653575

Gibbs, J. (2001). Maintaining front-line workers in child protection: A case for refocusing supervision. *Child Abuse Review, 10*, 323–335. doi:10.1002/ car.707

Gilbert, T. (2001). Reflective practice and clinical supervision: Meticulous rituals of the confessional. *Journal of Advanced Nursing, 36*(2), 199–205. https://doi.org/10.1046/j.1365-2648.2001.01960.x

Goddard, C., & Hunt, S. (2011). The complexities of caring for child protection workers: The contexts of practice and supervision. *Journal of Social Work Practice, 25*(4), 413–432. doi:10.1080/02650533.2011.626644

Harris, M., & Fallot, R. (2001). Envisioning a trauma informed service system: A vital paradigm shift. *New Directions for Mental Health Services, 89*, 3–22. doi:10.1002/yd.23320018903

Hunt, S., & Broadley, K. (2020). Education professionals' role in identifying and reporting child sexual abuse: Untangling the maze. In I. Bryce & W.

60   *Supervision*

Petherick (Eds.), *Child sexual abuse* (pp. 391–419). Academic Press. https://doi.org/10.1016/B978-0-12-819434-8.00019-2

Hunt, S., Goddard, C., Cooper, J., Littlechild, B., & Wild, J. (2016). 'If I feel like this, how does the child feel?' Child protection workers, supervision, management and organisational responses to parental violence. *Journal of Social Work Practice, 30*(1), 5–24. doi:10.1080/02650533.2015.1073145

Ingram, R. (2013). Emotions, social work practice and supervision: An uneasy alliance? *Journal of Social Work Practice, 27*(1), 5–19. https://doi.org/10.1080/02650533.2012.745842

Jankoski, J. (2010). Is vicarious trauma the culprit? A study of child welfare professionals. *Child Welfare, 89*(6), 105–131.

Johns, C. (2001). Depending on the intent and emphasis of the supervisor, clinical supervision can be a different experience. *Journal of Nursing Management, 9*(3), 139–145. https://doi.org/10.1046/j.1365-2834.2001.00208.x

Kadushin, A., & Harkness, D. (2014). *Supervision in social work* (5th ed.). Columbia University Press.

Kouzes, J., & Posner, B. (2016). Leading in cynical times. *Journal of Management Inquiry, 14*(4), 357–364. doi:10.1177/1056492605280221

Little, M., Baker, T., & Jinks, A. (2018). A qualitative evaluation of community nurses' experiences of child safeguarding supervision. *Child Abuse Review, 27*(2), 150–157. http://dx.doi.org/10.1002/car.2493.

NASW & ASWB. (2013). *Best practice standards in social work supervision.* NASW & ASWB.

Manthorpe, J., Moriarty, J., Hussein, S., Stevens, M., & Sharpe, E. (2015). Content and purpose of supervision in social work practice in England: Views of newly qualified social workers, managers and directors. *British Journal of Social Work, 45*(1), 52–68. doi:10.1093/bjsw/bct102

McCrae, J., Scannapieco, M., & Obermann, A. (2015). Retention and job satisfaction of child welfare supervisors. *Children and Youth Services Review, 59*, 171–176. doi:10.1016/j.childyouth.2015.11.011

McPherson, L., Frederico, M., & McNamara, P. (2016). Safety as a fifth dimension in supervision: Stories from the frontline. *Australian Social Work, 69*(1), 67–79. doi:10.1080/0312407X.2015.1024265

Morrison, T. (2001). *Staff supervision in social care: Making a real difference for staff and service users.* Pavilion.

Nickson, A., Carter, M., & Francis, A. (2019). *Supervision and professional development in social work practice.* Sage.

O'Donoghue, K. (2015). Issues and challenges facing social work supervision in the twenty-first century. *China Journal of Social Work, 8*(2), 136–149. doi:10.1080/17525098.2015.1039172

Oates, F. (2019). You are not allowed to tell: Organisational culture as a barrier for child protection workers seeking assistance for traumatic stress symptomology. *Children Australia, 44*(2), 84–90. doi:10.1017/cha.2019.12

Radey, M., & Stanley, L. (2018). "Hands on" versus "empty": Supervision experiences of frontline child welfare workers. *Children and Youth Services Review, 91*, 128–136. https://doi.org/10.1016/j.childyouth.2018.05.037

Rankine, M. (2019). The internal/external debate: The tensions within social work supervision. *Aotearoa New Zealand Social Work, 31*(3), 32–45. doi:10.11157/anzswj-vol31iss3id646

Regehr, C. (2018). *Stress, trauma, and decision-making for social workers.* Columbia University Press.

Substance Abuse and Mental Health Services Administration. (2014). *SAMHSA's concept of trauma and guidance for a trauma informed approach.* Substance Abuse and Mental Health Services Administration.

Tillman, K., Prazak, M., Burrier, L., Miller, S., Benezra, M., & Lynch, L. (2016). Factors influencing school counsellors suspecting and reporting of childhood physical abuse: Investigating child, parent, school, and abuse characteristics. *Professional School Counseling, 19*(1), 103–115. https://doi.org/10.5330/1096-2409-19.1.103

Tsang, N. (2006). Dialectics-the arts of teaching and learning in social work education. *Social Work Education, 25*(3), 265–278. https://doi.org/10.1080/02615470600565194

Tsui, M. (2005). *Social work supervision: Contexts and concepts.* Sage.

Wilkins, D., Forrester, D., & Grant, L. (2017). What happens in child and family social work supervision? *Child & Family Social Work, 22*(2), 942–951. doi:10.1111/cfs.12314

3   Managers and organisations

Introduction

As discussed already in this book, the practice settings in which professionals undertake work with vulnerable children and their families are vast. The kinds of professionals who have supervisory responsibility for practitioners working with these client groups are just as vast. It can often be the case that line managers responsible for providing direction and support to practitioners do not themselves have a practice background working with vulnerable children and their families. This happens for a number of reasons, including that managerial skills that are required to run big government-funded programs or programs run by large faith-based or charitable organisations are not typically taught in undergraduate or post-graduate human and health services degree programs. Another setting where this is prevalent is in the allied health sector, which is traditionally staffed by professionals from multi-disciplinary practice backgrounds.

In this chapter I explore the supervisory role within an organisational context, including barriers to providing effective supervision and support, the supervisory relationship between line managers and practitioners as well as the training, support and supervision needs of line supervisors and managers. Throughout the chapter are case studies and vignettes highlighting the complexities of undertaking a supervisory role in the practice contexts where services are delivered to vulnerable children and their families. For the purpose of clarity, no one narrative is a complete transcript of events. Rather, the narratives are a composition of my experience in practice, research and higher education contexts, demonstrating common challenges and dilemmas experienced by line supervisors and managers that have re-occurred during my involvement in the child protection service system.

DOI: 10.4324/9781003026006-4

The role of supervisors and managers in a child welfare context

Most organisations that provide services to vulnerable children and their families are funded either directly or indirectly by the government of the jurisdiction. Government-funded programs and services have strict contractual obligations attached to them which include detailed reporting. The structure of Government-provided services are by their nature structured hierarchically. In a general sense, line supervisors and managers of practitioners who work in this field constitute middle management, that is, a layer of management that exists between those who provide front-line services and the executive level of operations. Who makes up these layers will of course vary between jurisdictions.

While it is acknowledged that the practice settings and professional backgrounds of line supervisors and managers vary, the scope of the role is fairly consistent across jurisdictions. The duties undertaken by line supervisors and managers typically include all human resources (HR) matters including leave, timesheets and entitlements, the management of team workloads, and compliance with organisational and/ or legislative requirements. Some roles also include the management of budgets, key performance indicators and staff recruitment. Many line supervisors and managers are 'on call' for emergencies after normal business hours and on weekends.

The role in a multi-disciplinary context

As mentioned in previous chapters, practice settings where practitioners work with vulnerable children and their families vary widely. So do the role, scope and professional backgrounds of line supervisors and managers. As an example, a social worker working in a large state-run health care setting may have a line supervisor with a nursing or other allied health professional background. This is common in health care settings where multidisciplinary teams are the norm. However, many allied health undergraduate training programs do not include any learning material related to child abuse and neglect, leaving individuals to identify and remedy gaps in their own knowledge base. Another example may be a practitioner attached to a legal practice that works in the child and family area of law. Line supervisors in these settings are most often lawyers and in some cases human resource and office managers. In these examples, a lack of foundational knowledge regarding working with vulnerable children and their families can be a barrier to line supervisors and managers providing effective supervision to teams. The other barrier which must be acknowledged is that some professions don't routinely engage in supervision in the same way that the social work or psychology professions might, resulting in some line supervisors' first experience of supervision to be when they are required to provide it.

Case study: multidisciplinary teams

I manage a multidisciplinary team of professionals in a large health setting. I am a nurse by training however have been in health administration and management roles for 16 years. The team I supervise has social workers, nurses, occupational and speech therapists as well as psychologists on it. The part I struggle with most if I am honest is the emotional needs of the staff. They don't see child abuse every second of every day in their roles but when they do it is really bad. When we see child abuse it is usually due to a child experiencing significant injuries requiring a stay in hospital. The cause is most often physical or sexual abuse but can also be prolonged neglect. I tell them their job is to take care of that child and to move on to the next patient which some of them struggle with. They also get upset when child protection authorities come and take babies shortly after birth. I mean I am old school in a way – child welfare officers are doing what they need to, right? Those kids are better off in foster care. I know it's tough but I am not their therapist. I've got my own work to do.

A key duty of line supervisors and managers is of course, the support and supervision needs of practitioners working under them. However, what that looks like can vary widely between practice settings and individual line supervisors and managers. Line supervisors and managers often struggle with the dual roles of supervising practitioners and managing the performance of their teams overall. Balancing the role of managing and nurturing staff with the requirements of executives above them can be extremely challenging. The preceding example demonstrates these challenges.

The case study also demonstrates difficulties experienced by line supervisors and managers who may have some gaps in their foundational knowledge of child abuse and neglect. A child's experience of abuse and neglect does not happen independent of other societal and socio-political factors. Factors such as poverty, discrimination, intergenerational trauma and poor access to health, education, housing and employment are all underlying causes of child abuse and neglect.

Without this foundational knowledge, line supervisors and managers can struggle to provide informed support and professional counsel to supervisees.

As discussed in the supervision chapter, there is a strong argument for external supervision to be made available to practitioners as a mechanism to better address matters pertaining to wellbeing. This case study strengthens the rationale for professionals to engage in external supervision, not only for wellbeing matters but for professional content development as well. External supervision for line supervisors and managers where professional knowledge could be expanded would benefit them as well as the teams they manage.

Support for line supervisors and managers

There is a moderate level of research literature available that seeks to identify what professionals working with vulnerable children and their families need to increase job satisfaction, rates of retention and to support their wellbeing in the workplace. Many of these studies are critical of the role of the supervisor, often presenting supervisors in the same category of findings that pertain to senior executives in the organisation. The experiences of line supervisors are often not distinguished from frontline workers with no line management responsibility in the research literature. This of course fails to recognise that many line supervisors and managers are themselves experienced child welfare workers or child welfare administrators with unique support needs.

In a study of 111 child welfare supervisors in the United States, McCrae et al. (2015) found there was some correlation between previous studies focused on case workers and their study focused on supervisors, however there were also distinct differences. McCrae et al. (2015) found a correlation between supervisors experiencing high levels of job stress with an increased intention to leave their position which is consistent with studies by Hunt et al. (2016) which focused on frontline workers. However, when compared, McCrae et al. (2015) found that factors like perceived level of organisational support to be less of a determining factor for supervisors intending to leave.

As mentioned previously, organisational policies and procedures regarding the type and frequency of supervision practitioners are entitled to can vary widely across jurisdictions. As an example, frontline practitioners working in statutory child protection organisations almost universally have mandatory internal supervision requirements. Conversely, nurses across jurisdictions who work with children who

have experienced abuse and neglect typically don't have requirements for mandated internal supervision.

Supervision entitlements for line supervisors and managers tend
to be even more varied. In my own research, line supervisors and
managers who worked for non-government organisations that delivered services to vulnerable children and their families were most
likely to be entitled to ongoing external supervision funded by their
organisation. Line supervisors and managers who had worked in
statutory child protection agencies on the whole reported either
never receiving supervision or receiving only task-focused supervision. Some reported being able to access external supervision at
their own cost. McCrae et al.'s (2015) study found that child welfare
supervisors did not receive adequate supervision or support. McCrae
et al. (2015) cite that line supervisors who received adequate professional support would be more likely to successfully manage the
unique dynamics of their role and thus more effectively manage
their teams.

Also noteworthy is the way in which increases to frontline staffing
occur. Significant increases in frontline staffing often occur as a result
of a negative impetus, that is, the death or serious non-accidental
injury of a child and/or a resulting government-led inquiry into the
actions or non-actions of statutory child protection authorities. More
often than not, governments commit to increasing frontline staff as
a result. However, increases are seldom allocated to line supervisor
or manager positions. The unintended consequences of increases to
frontline staff are that the workloads of supervisors increase significantly without any additional resourcing, increasing pressure on middle management positions consistently over time.

Training and mentoring for line supervisors and managers

There is a moderate amount of research pertaining to the training
and mentoring needs of practitioners wishing to progress to management positions. The research literature regarding the upskilling of
practitioners into leadership positions cites a lack of emphasis at the
undergraduate level of the skills and knowledge required (Knee &
Folsom, 2012; Peters, 2018) and that practitioners can find themselves managing teams of people without relevant qualifications,
skills or experience (Carpenter et al., 2013; Hair, 2013; Kadushin &
Harkness, 2014). The lack of leadership training afforded to line

supervisors and managers particularly in relation to supporting the wellbeing needs of practitioners working in trauma-laden environments is noted in the practice research literature (Berger & Quiros, 2014; Goddard & Hunt, 2011; Jankoski, 2010). Research undertaken by McCrae et al. (2015) clearly outlines that it is critical that line supervisors and managers receive regular quality supervision to support them in their roles.

Anecdotally, there are limited or poorly defined pathways for practitioners wishing to progress to line management positions across a number of jurisdictions. For example, practitioners viewed by line managers as having leadership potential are 'shoulder tapped' to backfill the permanent line manager for short periods while they go on annual leave. Practitioners undertaking these backfill positions often still carry their own caseload in addition to their new managerial duties, leaving little time for upskilling or critical reflection. Practitioners who undertake periodic management stints can find themselves moving into more permanent management roles without adequate qualifications, mentoring or ongoing training.

Case study: transition from practitioner to line supervisor

After a while working as a frontline case manager, I wanted to progress to a line manager position. When my own line manager went on maternity leave, I was asked to backfill her role – what a baptism by fire! I had no idea what managing people was actually going to be like – no one tells you what it's really like until you are in the role and managing all sorts of staff-related dramas – complaints, performance management, unprofessional conduct, grievances between staff, crisis within the personal lives of staff impacting them at work – it never ended! I had no idea and was really unprepared.

I have previously discussed the reluctance of practitioners to disclose their struggles with occupational traumatic stress to line supervisors and managers for fear of negative consequences like reducing a practitioner's likelihood of progressing to more senior positions. It is my view that this fear can be more pronounced among line supervisors and managers. The 'sink or swim' culture within workplaces that often precedes a practitioner's ability to progress to more senior positions does ingrain unrealistic workload expectations and an environment where asking questions risks a practitioner being seen as not cut out for management.

*Case study: support and supervision needs as a line supervisor
or manager*

*When I was a case worker, the thing I valued most about supervision was
getting direction with where I should be going with families on my case
list. I would never have talked about my own stuff with my line supervisor – I am not that kind of person to share personal stuff and I don't
think my supervisor at the time was either. They never offered and I never
asked. But now that I am a supervisor of caseworkers I find myself really
struggling. There is so much more to this role than I thought. I find myself
constantly overwhelmed by the needs of my staff, the needs of the kids, the
needs of my organisation – it's constant worry and I feel like I am drown-
ing but I feel I can't really tell anyone. I know if I stumble or show weak-
ness there are 10 more people waiting to take my job.*

The 'sink or swim' organisational culture, coupled with inconsistent supervision policies, can create an environment that further
isolates line supervisors and managers from seeking responsive
support that acknowledges their unique position in child welfare
organisations.

Although formal pathways to leadership may vary between organisations and jurisdictions, there are some examples of how individual
line supervisors and managers can informally mentor practitioners
who demonstrate a desire to progress to leadership positions.

Case study: good professional support experiences

*When I finished university I knew I wanted to work in child protection.
My first manager was so wonderful, I really admired her and wanted to
be just like her. She was warm and I felt comfortable telling her that eventually I would like to manage my own team. Once I had told her that, she
started to mentor me in the job – we came up with a professional development plan – nothing too detailed, but things like when appropriate she
would take me to various meetings so I could observe how she managed
tense meetings with clients as well as with stakeholders internally and
externally. She also engaged me in conversations that were broader than
just my cases while in supervision – things like balancing organisational
requirements, budgets, etc., with best practice interventions with clients
and how to work through those issues when they clash with each other.
I have been in leadership positions now for about 10 years and I still
value that period of time when she took me under her wing. I still hear
her voice in my head now!*

As this case study demonstrates, informal pathways can be just as impactful as formal training opportunities.

Line supervisor and manager experience of occupational trauma, including stressors

Throughout the research literature, line supervisors and managers tend to receive much of the criticism in relation to organisational failure to provide practitioners with adequate resources and supports, including supervision. However, it is often not stated that line supervisors and managers are exposed to the same occupational traumas as frontline child protection practitioners, often for longer periods of time, without professional support. Additionally, line supervisors and managers are exposed to what happens 'when things go wrong', as they are often the ones in witness stands and enquiries when a child has died or experienced a significant non-accidental injury at the hands of a caregiver. While this is an occupational stressor also experienced by frontline staff, the responsibility most often sits with line supervisors and managers, as do the consequences.

Another significant work related stressor experienced by line supervisors and managers is the management of unallocated work due to staff shortages. Further affecting line supervisors and managers is the ongoing impact of decision making delegation. In simplistic terms, it is often the decision of line supervisors and managers which child is more at risk and should be seen first, which child should be removed from their family's care to ensure their safety, which child should be returned to their family's care and which child goes into the unallocated 'work' pool in response to a lack of staff.

Case study: anxiety and unallocated work

I manage a team of child welfare workers. Our team manages statutory cases. The job is hard and we have a constant churn of staff. We always have more cases than case workers. The cases without allocated workers sit with me. All the families are high risk. It is impossible for me to know what is going on with each one. Anything could be happening to those kids. It keeps me awake at night. The anxiety of knowing something terrible could happen at any time is overwhelming if you think about it for too long.

Geoffrion et al. (2016) describe stress as a result of positional and professional accountability as an under-researched phenomenon experienced by professionals working in a child welfare context.

Another source of occupational distress for line supervisors and managers is the lack of empathy for the inherent difficulties of their positions both internally and externally to their organisation. Examples of this can be found during workplace injury negotiations or with unions, usually in relation to workloads. While it is often the case that line supervisors and managers have more onerous workloads than the practitioners they supervise, they are often the ones who find themselves having to justify practitioner workloads to external bodies, the resolution of which is often for them to take on more work. Line supervisors and managers are seldom in positions where they can effect change regarding allocation of resources; however, they are often in positions where they need to manage the outcomes of poor resource allocation decisions.

> *Case study: why I can't deliver the supervision*
> *needed to my staff*
>
> *I have been a supervisor of child welfare professionals for about 8 years. The part of supervising that I have found really stressful over time is that all your time gets spent managing things like care plan completion rates, budget allocations, complaints and other menial tasks. You never get the time to actually properly support your staff to do the work they need to do. I also carry all the unallocated work because we always have case worker vacancies. Staff can be needy at times, yes, but that's because they need emotional and practice support as well as administrative and procedural support. I just don't have the time. I wish I did but I just don't.*

Line supervisors and managers have to manage teams of practitioners under them as well as deal with higher-level management. As already discussed, there are many complex factors that contribute to a line supervisor's inability to provide quality supervision, many of which are outside of their control. However, being the 'meat in the sandwich' can make the position of line supervisor or manager a very isolated and lonely one.

> *Case study: promoted within the team*
>
> *As a frontline practitioner, I loved being a part of my team. I felt supported and valued as a team member. Then I took on the line manager position when it became vacant – my team mates who I had felt so connected to and who I relied on so heavily for professional support slowly started to pull away from me – I would stop getting invited for drinks,*

chatter would stop when I walked into the work area, people stopped sharing things with me – I guess they saw me as 'management' now – it was a very dislocating experience.

The initial and ongoing professional support needs of practitioners wishing to progress to line management positions is in my view an under-researched area that requires additional investigation.

Re-thinking the role of the supervisor

Now that we have explored the role and challenges of line supervisors and managers in the child welfare organisational context, it is my view that re-thinking the role of the supervisor, particularly in relation to the provision of supervision and support to practitioners, would be a useful endeavour. As mentioned in the previous chapter, there is consistent criticism in the literature about the inability of organisations to provide quality and responsive supervision to practitioners working with vulnerable children and their families. Key reasons for this identified in the literature include: organisational constraints like resourcing, internal organisational culture and negative perceptions held by practitioners about the purpose of supervision (Beddoe & Davys, 2016; Hunt et al., 2016; Oates, 2019). As outlined in the previous chapter, the quality of the supervisory relationship is a precursor to practitioners feeling supported in relation to practice and wellbeing matters, practitioners feeling professionally confident and practitioners staying longer in their positions. A number of studies have outlined that the positive professional relationship between practitioners and their supervisors is a key contributor to practitioner wellbeing and a protective measure against the ongoing experience of occupational traumatic stress (Davys & Beddoe, 2010; Pack, 2015).

Given the evidence that positive supervisory relationships correlate with practitioner wellbeing, increased levels of job satisfaction and increased practitioner retention, and the consistent criticism that organisations struggle to provide effective supervision, perhaps it is time to critically reflect on the role of the line supervisor. Should line supervisors be the primary source of support and supervision for practitioners working with vulnerable children and their families? Should they be primarily responsible for the induction and ongoing mentoring of new practitioners, particularly given their workloads? Is it ethical for line supervisors and managers to have the dual role of managing practitioner performance and being the central point for practitioners to access support for wellbeing issues? Would diffusing these critical roles to other modes of support be more beneficial for the practitioner? For the line supervisor?

The supervisory relationship from the perspective of the supervisor

In the previous chapter, I explored the role of the supervisor and the supervisory relationship from the perspective of the practitioner. In this chapter, I explore the supervisory relationship from the perspective of the supervisor. As previously mentioned, there is a dearth of research exploring the perspectives of line supervisors and managers who support practitioners working in trauma-laden environments.

Dilemmas in supervision: supervision or therapy?

One of the most common dilemmas experienced by line supervisors managing teams of professionals who work in trauma-laden environments is where supervision ends and therapy starts. Line supervisors and managers have the precarious position of supporting staff who may be struggling with their own experiences of trauma as well as managing the workload and performance of staff as already outlined in this chapter.

Managing practitioners with a lived experience of trauma

In my own research, practice experience and anecdotally, supervising practitioners with a lived experience of trauma, abuse and neglect is a common experience of line supervisors and managers and one that can create many complexities and ethical dilemmas for line supervisors and managers.

Case study: violent parent triggers practitioner's history of domestic and family violence

I was supervising a recent graduate when they were allocated a new family where the mother and father had separated – the child they shared went into out-of-home care. The father had strong gang ties and a significant criminal history. The mother had told initial investigating officers to be careful of her ex-partner as he had a propensity for violence, particularly toward figures of authority. Our agency was seeking a custody order for the child for 12 months. The caseworker assigned to the case started to become particularly avoidant when I would ask her about where the outstanding assessments for the father were at – this was important as there was a tight timeframe due to the ongoing court matter. She would brush me off, saying things were happening. She started to avoid supervision altogether and would spend most of her time out of the office. She had made arrangements for the outstanding assessments relating to the mother, however as the court date approached there was still no completed assessment relating to the father. In our jurisdiction, the supervisor is named as the respondent and presents the matter in court, even though the majority of the assessment work is completed by the caseworker. With the court deadline looming I had to insist that the caseworker make themselves available to give me an update. She broke down in my office stating that she was overwhelmed with the case and that she was fearful of having contact with the father due to his aggressive and demeaning behaviour towards her. She said she had not been sleeping and that she was paralysed with anxiety when she thought of having to speak with the father. She said the father reminded her of her own violent ex-partner and that she was having flashbacks from when she was still in that relationship. She said she would be going to the doctor for a certificate to take extended sick leave as she was not coping. I was shocked by this. And also angry. And disappointed. Dealing with unpleasant parents is a part of the job – why didn't they tell me before the court date so I could plan around it? I then had to pull overtime to complete this work on top of my already bursting workload. I didn't get home in time to see my own children before they went to bed all of that next week. Looking back, I feel like I could have been more attentive and then maybe I would have seen the avoidant behaviour as a sign she was struggling – but I also had 6 other staff to look after plus my own workload – surely she had a responsibility to manage her own wellbeing as well? I still feel conflicted about it.

This case study demonstrates the complexities experienced by line supervisors and managers who have the dual role of managing the wellbeing of practitioners, the workloads of the team and their own workload. These situations are extremely common, and as the case study demonstrates, there is often no clear best practice to manage them.

Supervising practitioners who have a history of childhood trauma is common and can leave line supervisors and managers unsure of how to most effectively support those practitioners. This is especially relevant when a practitioner's experience of childhood trauma appears to be directly negatively affecting a practitioner's ability to undertake their paid duties.

Case study: practitioners with lived experience

I was managing a team of practitioners who worked with vulnerable children and young people that were in the care of the statutory child protection authority. A new worker started who initially I was pleased about because she had had some experience working with young people in out of home care and I thought I wouldn't have to spend a lot of time inducting her. Very early she started displaying what I thought was unusual behaviour. She seemed over familiar with me and other members of the team. She seemed almost manic at times and didn't pick up on the cues from the team that her over-the-top, over familiar behaviour wasn't welcome. As the weeks went by it seemed very evident that she had formed relationships with the young people on their case list and was spending time with them outside of her paid work hours. I brought her in to address these issues. In the session she told me that she came from a dysfunctional family of origin and that whilst she was never taken into the care of the state, she felt that she should have been. She said that her childhood experience of abuse and neglect is what drew her to the work and that she had a special understanding of what the young people on her caseload were experiencing. She stated that she could not understand why spending time with the young people outside of her paid hours was inappropriate – she stated that if someone would have invested extra time in her when she was younger, she may not have experienced some of the trauma she did. She said that the 'cold hands off' approach with traumatised young people was the problem with the system and that she was going to be different. I of course had to start a performance management process with her. I couldn't trust her to work unsupervised. I spent so much time managing this one worker I completely neglected the others. On reflection I could have managed the situation better – maybe I should have referred her to therapy? On the other hand, she's an adult and I really don't think that's my role.

This case study demonstrates the experience of many line supervisors and managers who feel unsure of how to manage these complexities. Supervisors struggling to define where their role as supervisor ends and the role of therapist begins are discussed in the literature by authors such as Pendry (2012), Graves (2008) and Wheeler (2007). Wheeler (2007) wrote that:

> the extent to which supervisors should offer therapeutic support to supervisees is debatable . . . supervision is not about therapy . . . ways in which the well-being of a counsellor impacts on the client . . . must be addressed . . . a balance needs to be

struck that enables exploration and support, but avoids supervision as therapy.

(pp. 246–247)

In addition to line supervisors and managers being unsure of how to manage staff who have histories of childhood trauma, there are times when they themselves may struggle to put their own lived experiences aside in order for them to best support practitioners.

Case study: I can, why can't they?

I had a case worker start and on their first day they announced that they wouldn't work with violent parents – men or women – because they had a history of childhood trauma. I mean, I didn't grow up in the most functional of families either, there was a lot of violence in our house – but I have managed to deal with it and put those issues aside while I am at work – why can't they? Most of the families known to us have some level of violence present – what am I meant to do? Not allocate any cases to them? Some people just aren't cut out for this work.

As previously outlined, McCrae et al. (2015) write that the provision of quality supervision to line supervisors and managers should be a central practice of organisations. The case study here demonstrates that good quality supervision that provides an opportunity for line supervisors and managers to critically reflect on their own histories of trauma and how that may be affecgting their management of teams is consistent with the work of McCrae et al. (2015).

Practitioner's lived experience as an asset

It must be acknowledged that managing the wellbeing support needs of practitioners can be difficult for line supervisors and managers for a myriad of reasons. However, it must also be acknowledged that practitioners with lived experience can be assets to organisations who work with vulnerable children and their families. In the research literature, Newcomb et al. (2015) discuss the concept of the wounded healer, an archetype used by Jung, to describe the position of people in the healing professions who themselves have a personal history of trauma. There is some consensus in the literature that practitioners who have a lived experience of trauma can possess qualities that complement their professional skills and knowledge, like increased empathy and ability to work with complexity (Wheeler, 2007; Zerubavel & Wright,

2012). Conversely, there are views cited in the literature that without appropriate organisational support, practitioners with lived experience of trauma are at risk of being viewed by their organisation in a negative light due to the demonstration of negative 'wounded healer' attributes (Guggenbuhl-Craig, 1999; Zerubavel & Wright, 2012).

As discussed previously, there is an established evidence base indicating that organisations that deliver services to vulnerable children and their families often have an internal culture that dissuades practitioners from disclosing either their own history of trauma or a developed experience of occupational trauma and openly seeking assistance to manage these wellbeing issues (Goddard & Hunt, 2011; Hunt et al., 2016; Oates, 2019). This organisational culture of non-disclosure acts as a barrier for many practitioners seeking timely support for trauma-related symptomology. In relation to organisational support for practitioners with a history of trauma, Zerubavel and Wright (2012) argue for 'the fundamental importance of having disclosure as a viable option for wounded healers in need of support'. They continue:

> It is problematic if our profession has developed an atmosphere in which it is stigmatising to acknowledge vulnerability or woundedness . . . such a milieu puts wounded healers at greater risk of unaddressed impairment by precluding opportunities to assess the impact of woundedness and to suggest intervention when needed.
>
> (p. 487)

Wheeler (2007) argued that 'while the supervisor cannot be the therapist, the personal life of the [practitioner] cannot be ignored . . . supervisors have an important role to play in recognising and attending to the wounds of the healer' (p. 255). Although in agreement, Berger and Quiros (2016) acknowledge that:

> while supervising any practitioner with a personal trauma history is challenging, working in trauma-impacted environments where encountering traumatised clients is consistent and extensive is a significant risk factor for triggering vicarious re-traumatisation and thus requires particular attention . . . shying away from this discussion in supervision may compromise the necessary depth of understanding the multifaceted nature of trauma and ultimately impact both the therapeutic alliance and the accompanying individual and group interventions.
>
> (p. 151)

While there is a lack of consensus regarding the role and boundaries of the supervisor in relation to the management of wellbeing matters in supervision, what is clear is that the experience of occupational traumatic stress is an occupational inevitability. Given this, it would be my recommendation that all practitioners working in trauma-laden environments with vulnerable children and their families be seen through the lens of the wounded healer architype. With that lens in place, the provision of responsive support for practitioners and line supervisors may become somewhat clearer.

Line supervision and management within a child welfare organisational context: the rise of managerialism

So far in this chapter we have explored the role and specific challenges of the line supervisor and manager in a support and supervision context. Now I will expand outwards and take a macro look at organisational contexts, including organisational cultures present within workplaces that provide services to vulnerable children and families and how the line supervisor and manager role is located in this context. Authors like Beddoe and Davys (2016) and Hughes and Wearing (2017) acknowledge that the roles taken on by human services professionals, including their practice, are often defined or prescribed by the employing organisation. Exploring organisational impacts on practice is therefore necessary. Drumm (2012) defines organisational culture as embodiment of 'shared values, beliefs and assumptions that are deeply ingrained in an organisation's traditions, and influence how an organisation thinks and feels' (p. 1).

One of the greatest organisational, operational, practice and cultural changes to occur within human and social service delivery over the past few decades has been the rise of managerialism. Managerialism is an outcome of Western governments shifting to an ideological position of neoliberalism. The tenets of neoliberalism heavily rely on the principles of the market to inform operational policy and practice (Ferguson & Lavalette, 2013). An example of what this looks like in a human and social services context is the outsourcing of services previously provided directly by governments, e.g., family support services, disability support and employment services (Carey, 2015; Hughes & Wearing, 2017). Organisations relying on short-term contracts, casual workers and labour-hire companies to provide staff are also examples of organisational practices consistent with neoliberal ideologies. Another visible outcome of moving human services organisations to a mangerialistic focus are the seemingly never-ending efficiency reviews, restructures and rebranding, most of which have very little to do with the actual delivery of services that are core business (Carey, 2015).

Managerialism is identified in the literature as a barrier to providing practitioners with the support and supervision they require to effectively perform their roles in the child protection workplace (Beddoe, 2012; Hughes & Wearing, 2017; Noble & Irwin, 2009). In the neoliberal context, social and human services organisations that are government run and government funded view themselves as the deliverer or sub-contractor of services. That is their core business, their core purpose. Missing in the neoliberal ideology is an organisation's responsibility to support, develop and nurture the professionals delivering those services. Increasingly, especially in climates of austerity, if a practitioner is not receiving the support and supervision they require internally, then it is the practitioner who is responsible for seeking out additional supports rather than the organisation taking responsibility and reviewing the quality and responsiveness of the support they offer to practitioners in their employ.

Case study: supervision external to a practitioner's organisation

I have worked with vulnerable children and families for 12 years, 5 of those years in a line manager position. I know I can't provide the best supervision to the team because of all the competing priorities I have to manage. When new staff start, I tell them to get external supervision in their own time and claim the fees back on their tax as a professional education expense. Realistically, that's the only way they are going to get that kind of professional support.

In the literature, there is some debate about the way in which supervision is viewed by organisations in a managerialist context. Hughes and Wearing (2017) contend that managerialism is fuelled by economic and political agendas that tend to be external to the core business of organisations. This can result in the role of human and social service practitioners being determined by these ideological underpinnings rather than by evidence-based best practice. Another example, outlined in the literature by Beddoe (2012), demonstrates how mangerialism can alter the way supervision is viewed by organisations that work with vulnerable children and their families. Beddoe (2012) discusses in the literature that organisations can view supervision as a 'vaccine against mistakes' rather than a process of supporting the professional wellbeing and development of practitioners (p. 201). Noble and Irwin (2009) also discuss the way that managerialist climates within organisations have facilitated a shift back towards supervision that is administrative and compliance driven, rather than a process of professional development for practitioners. This is despite clear evidence-based research that heavily administrative and compliance-driven supervision does not adequately meet the support and development needs of practitioners who work with vulnerable children and their families.

Management and leadership in a child welfare organisational context

Now that we have looked at mangerialism as a key influence within the way human and social service organisations operate, I will explore how organisational influences affects leadership. There is consistent criticism in the literature about poor management practices in organisations that work with vulnerable children and their families. Further, poor management practices are identified in the literature as a risk to the wellbeing of practitioners, among them the lack of access to quality support and supervision (Hunt et al., 2016; Oates, 2019). Peters (2018) contends that in the absence of social service–specific leadership models, social welfare organisations have relied on management frameworks commonly used in business and other hierarchical institutions like the defence forces. These management models are characterised as being transactional in nature rather than relational, which can be at odds with most contemporary human service practice frameworks (Lawler & Bilson, 2013; Peters, 2018). As an example, transactional management models may view practitioners as resources that can be made more productive if efficiency measures are implemented, whereas a relational model of management would view practitioners, particularly those who work directly with clients, as assets with expertise that should be valued and invested in.

The viewing of practitioners as replaceable resources (an operational cost that efficiency measures can be applied to) rather than assets (holders of knowledge and expertise related to core business), creates an organisational environment that makes it difficult for practitioners to contribute their expertise to inform critical reflection and organisational change that may be systemic in nature. These top-down styles of management have been shown to be problematic in a human and social services context as practitioners are not units of stock and vulnerable children and families are not liabilities to efficiency

(Hughes & Wearing, 2017). Further change should be informed by evidence-based practice and evaluation, not by the forces that are central to neo-liberal and managerialist ideology (Ferguson & Lavalette, 2013).

Top-down neo-liberal ideology within organisations that provide services to vulnerable children and their families is problematic, especially in the context of supporting the professional development and wellbeing of practitioners. Hughes and Wearing (2017), drawing on transformational leadership practice, argue that line supervisors and managers within child protection organisations should view themselves as a 'manager of meaning' instead of a 'director of tasks' (pp. 125–126). Supporting practitioners to view themselves, their concerns and struggles within a larger system locates their professional and personal distress outside of themselves and within the structures that support contemporary child welfare service delivery. This strategy is critical for line supervisors and managers to integrate into their support and supervision practice with practitioners and is a practical strategy that facilitates a practitioner's ability to move through occupational traumatic stress symptomology. Given that we have established that the experience of occupational trauma is an occupational inevitability for practitioners working with vulnerable children and their families, organisational leadership frameworks that are attuned to trauma informed principles would be most appropriate.

Trauma informed and responsive leadership

The framework underpinning any trauma informed practice, leadership practice or otherwise, must be informed by the six trauma informed principles namely, safety; trustworthiness and transparency; peer support; collaboration and mutuality; empowerment, voice and choice; and cultural, historical and gender considerations (SAMHSA, 2014). These principles were introduced in previous chapters and will be explored in more detail in coming chapters. Trauma-responsive leadership occurs when staff employed by an organisation experience empathy, understanding and compassion towards their clients and their staff. Practitioners working in organisations with a trauma informed leadership framework would ideally feel safe, respected, valued and recognised for their knowledge and expertise. Trauma informed leadership can happen only in a truly trauma informed organisation. A trauma informed organisational response is underpinned by a relational approach, namely, a cyclical process of learning and support from top down and bottom up.

As previously presented in this book, SAMHSA (2014) outlined that trauma informed organisations must be underpinned by four key elements: realisation, recognition, response, and resist. These are commonly referred to in the literature as the four Rs. Wall et al. (2016, p. 9) summarise the four Rs as:

1. *Realisation* at all levels of an organisation or system about trauma and its impacts on individuals, families and communities;
2. *Recognition* of the signs of trauma;
3. *Response* – program, organisation or system responds by applying the principles of a trauma informed approach; and
4. *Resist* re-traumatisation of clients as well as staff.

It is my view that the four Rs could be applied by line supervisors and managers to better support the professional wellbeing of frontline practitioners. As an example, the outsourcing of some practitioner supervision and support functions would in my view be a demonstration of trauma informed leadership. While I acknowledge that funding external supervision for large numbers of staff would be prohibitive due to the cost, a solution may be to fund a specialist position to provide these services. Locating that position outside of the organisation, perhaps in a co-location scenario, would assist with perceived alignment with a practitioner's organisation and would reduce suspicion that confidentiality would not be adhered to.

Secure base leadership

Transactional leadership and trauma informed leadership frameworks are not the only frameworks identified in the literature as being well suited to organisations that provide services to vulnerable children and their families. Secure base leadership is a concept developed by George Kohlrieser, a clinical and organisational psychologist. The central tenet of secure base leadership is about creating a space where practitioners feel safe, supported and in control. These safe bases support practitioners to move through stressful and traumatic situations that arise as part of their work with vulnerable children and their families. This process of moving through occupational traumatic stress successfully builds an internal sense of resilience in practitioners and confidence that the next time a traumatic situation occurs, they have the skills to manage.

It must be acknowledged, however, that the concept of resilience is often discussed in the literature in a negative light. The concept of resilience is commonly referred to in the literature as being an innate quality possessed only by competent practitioners, with the underlying assumption being that those who have resilience will not be affected by occupational trauma. The acquisition of 'resilience' is cited as a solution to managing practitioners who are experiencing occupational traumatic stress. Practitioners who are significantly affected by occupational traumatic stress are described in the resilience literature as lacking the innate quality and therefore are perhaps not well suited to working in trauma-laden environments. This definition of resilience is not the same as the desired outcome of secure base leadership. Secure base leadership acknowledges that occupational traumatic stress is an inevitability, the management of which is an ongoing process. Secure base leadership fosters an environment where practitioners can safely process difficult occupational experiences, increasing their capacity to face occupationally difficult situations from a position of internal safety. Practitioners who operate from a space of internal safety are better placed to assess risk to vulnerable children and their families as their ability to identify and process information is less likely to be interrupted by their own sense of threat. Operating from a base of safety is also key for line supervisors and managers. When line supervisors and managers have good regulation of their own reactions to practitioner distress, moving those practitioners back to their own internal base of safety and security can be achieved more successfully. The ability to guide practitioners through an occupationally difficult experience back to a base of internal safety is a key outcome of secure base leadership and is consistent with the tenets of trauma informed and responsive leadership frameworks.

Chapter summary

In this chapter we have explored the role of line supervisors and managers in an occupational and organisational context. The support and training needs have been discussed and the lack of formal pathways available to practitioners wishing to move into a management position has been identified. Unique occupational traumas experienced by line supervisors and managers were identified and potential impacts on teams were discussed. The supervisory relationship from the perspective of line supervisors and managers was explored, supplemented by case studies that demonstrate common dilemmas experienced by line supervisors and managers. The rise of managerialism within human and social service organisations was discussed, as were leadership frameworks.

Reflective practice questions

1. As a supervisor, what would assist your professional development and wellbeing needs?
2. Is it ethical to have a line supervisor with the dual role of professional support and workload management? If not, what might some alternatives be in your workplace?
3. As a line supervisor or manager, how would you develop a secure base for the practitioners you supervise?

References

Beddoe, L. (2012). External supervision in social work: Power, space, risk, and the search for safety. *Australian Social Work, 65*(2), 197–213. https://doi.org/10.1080/0312407X.2011.591187

Beddoe, L., & Davys, A. (2016). *Challenges in professional supervision: Current themes and models for practice.* Jessica Kingsley Publishers.

Berger, R., & Quiros, L. (2014). Supervision for trauma informed practice. *Traumatology: An International Journal, 20*(4), 296–301. doi:10.1037/h0099835

Berger, R., & Quiros, L. (2016). Best practices for training trauma informed practitioners: Supervisors' voice. *Traumatology, 22*(2), 145–154. doi:10.1037/trm0000076

Carey, M. (2015). The fragmentation of social work and social care: Some ramifications and a critique. *British Journal of Social Work, 45*(8), 2406–2422. doi:10.1093/bjsw/bcu088

Carpenter, J., Webb, C., & Bostock, L. (2013). The surprisingly weak evidence base for supervision: Findings from a systematic review of research in child welfare practice (2000–2012). *Children and Youth Services Review, 35*(11), 1843–1853. https://doi.org/10.1016/j.childyouth.2013.08.014

Davys, A., & Beddoe, L. (2010). *Best practice in professional supervision: A guide for the helping professions.* Jessica Kingsley.

Drumm, M. (2012). *Culture change in the public sector.* https:// www.iriss.org.uk/resources/insights/culture-change-public-sector

Ferguson, I., & Lavalette, M. (2013). Crisis, austerity and the future(s) of social work in the UK. *Critical and Radical Social Work, 1*(1), 95–110. doi:10.1332/204986013X665992

Geoffrion, S., Morselli, C., & Guay, S. (2016). Rethinking compassion fatigue through the lens of professional identity: The case of child-protection workers. *Trauma, Violence & Abuse, 17*(3), 270–283. https://doi.org/10.1177/1524838015584362

Goddard, C., & Hunt, S. (2011). The complexities of caring for child protection workers: The contexts of practice and supervision. *Journal of Social Work Practice, 25*(4), 413–432. doi:10.1080/02650533.2011.626644

Graves, L. (2008). Teaching the wounded healer. *Medical Teacher, 30*(2), 217–219. doi:10.1080/01421590801948034

Guggenbuhl-Craig, A. (1999). *Power in the helping professions.* Spring Publications.

Hair, H. (2013). The purpose and duration of supervision, and the training and discipline of supervisors: What social workers say they need to provide effective services. *The British Journal of Social Work, 43,* 1562–1588. http://dx.doi.org/10.1093/ bjsw/bcs071

Hughes, M., & Wearing, M. (2017). *Organisations and management in social work: Everyday action for change* (3rd ed.). Sage.

Hunt, S., Goddard, C., Cooper, J., Littlechild, B., & Wild, J. (2016). 'If I feel like this, how does the child feel?' Child protection workers, supervision, management and organisational responses to parental violence. *Journal of Social Work Practice, 30*(1), 5–24. doi:10.1080/02650533.2015.1073145

Jankoski, J. (2010). Is vicarious trauma the culprit? A study of child welfare professionals. *Child Welfare, 89*(6), 105–131.

Kadushin, A., & Harkness, D. (2014). *Supervision in social work* (5th ed.). Columbia University Press.

Knee, R., & Folsom, J. (2012). Bridging the crevasse between direct practice social work and management by increasing the transferability of core skills. *Administration in Social Work, 36,* 390–408. doi:10.1080/03643107.2011. 604402

Lawler, J., & Bilson, A. (2013). *Social work management and leadership: Managing complexity with creativity.* Routledge.

McCrae, J., Scannapieco, M., & Obermann, A. (2015). Retention and job satisfaction of child welfare supervisors. *Children and Youth Services Review, 59,* 171–176. doi:10.1016/j.childyouth.2015.11.011

Newcomb, M., Burton, J., Edwards, N., & Hazelwood, Z. (2015). How Jung's concept of the wounded healer can guide learning and teaching in social work and human services. *Advances in Social Work and Welfare Education, 17*(2), 55–69.

Noble, C., & Irwin, J. (2009). Social work supervision: An exploration of the current challenges in a rapidly changing social, economic and political environment. *Journal of Social Work, 9*(3), 345–358. doi:10.1177/1468017309 334848

Oates, F. (2019). You are not allowed to tell: Organisational culture as a barrier for child protection workers seeking assistance for traumatic stress symptomology. *Children Australia, 44*(2), 84–90. doi:10.1017/cha.2019.12

Pack, M. (2015). 'Unsticking the stuckness': A qualitative study of the clinical supervisory needs of early-career health social workers. *British Journal of Social Work, 45*(6), 1821–1836. doi:10.1093/bjsw/bcu069

Pendry, N. (2012). Race, racism and systemic supervision. *Journal of Family Therapy, 34*(4), 403–418. doi:10.1111/j.1467-6427.2011.00576.x

Peters, S. (2018). Defining social work leadership: A theoretical and conceptual review and analysis. *Journal of Social Work Practice, 32*(1), 31–44. https://doi.org/10.1080/02650533.2017.1300877

Substance Abuse and Mental Health Services Administration. (2014). *SAMHSA's concept of trauma and guidance for a trauma informed approach.* Substance Abuse and Mental Health Services Administration.

Wall, L., Higgins, D., & Hunter, C. (2016). *Trauma informed care in child/family welfare services* (CFCA Paper No. 37). Child Family Community Australia Information Exchange, Australian Institute of Family Studies.

Wheeler, S. (2007). What shall we do with the wounded healer? The supervisor's dilemma. *Psychodynamic Practice, 13*(3), 245–256. doi:10.1080/14753630701455838

Zerubavel, N., & Wright, M. (2012). The dilemma of the wounded healer. *Psychotherapy, 49*(4), 482–491. doi:10.1037/a0027824

4 The TISS model

Introduction: what is the TISS model?

As discussed throughout this book, it is clear from the research literature that traditional internal methods of supervision consistently do
not meet the needs of practitioners who work with vulnerable children and their families. There are legitimate reasons for the lack of
effectiveness of internal support and supervision, including onerous
workloads, reduction in available funding for staff support and the
continued rise of managerialism – all of which have been discussed
previously in this book. Continued attempts to remedy the barriers
that hinder practitioner access to internal professional support and
supervision should continue. However, advocacy for improvement by
organisations as a sole strategy has been largely unsuccessful, creating
the rationale for alternative models to be considered.

At the core of the TISS model are the practitioners themselves.
Throughout this book, it has been established that working with vulnerable children and their families is some of the most complex work
practitioners can undertake in the human and social services sector.
The work is trauma-laden in nature and a practitioner will inevitably
experience occupational traumatic stress. This evidence base underpins
the TISS model in that it acknowledges that practitioners require both
ongoing professional development and wellbeing support to be successful in their roles. The TISS model also acknowledges that effective and
ongoing professional development and wellbeing support cannot be
solely provided by a practitioner's individual line supervisor or manager.

Principles underpinning the TISS model

Forming the basis of the TISS model are the six trauma informed
principles already outlined in this book. Those six principles are

DOI: 10.4324/9781003026006-5

safety; trustworthiness and transparency; peer support; collaboration and mutuality; empowerment, voice and choice; and cultural, historical and gender considerations (SAMHSA, 2014). Overarching the six trauma informed principles is the tenet that creating safety in the supervisory relationship is critical. Safety in relationships and processes within a supervision context reduces the threat response that practitioners may experience, especially those who have had negative experiences with supervision in the past. They also form the foundation from which practitioners can critically reflect on their practice as well as their own wellbeing and professional development. I will now discuss each of these six principles, how they inform the TISS model and how they can be applied in practice.

Safety: the safety principle applied within the TISS model context can refer to a practitioner's sense of safety within the supervisory relationship, both perceived and actual. The literature on practitioner experience of supervision has found that some practitioners avoid engaging in meaningful supervision due to a view that supervision is a tool used by their organisation to surveil them and their work. The safety principle can also underpin a practitioner's decision to share matters pertaining to their wellbeing.

Trustworthiness and transparency: the trustworthiness and transparency principle in the TISS model can refer to a shared sense of trust between a practitioner and their supervisor. As mentioned previously, the building and maintenance of trust in the supervisory relationship is critical and has been identified in the research literature as a key factor in a practitioner's ability to move through traumatic occupational experiences. The transparency part of this element should refer to transparency within the supervision process, that is, having clarity on the purpose of supervision, why certain matters are discussed and what the information will and will not be used for.

Peer support: The peer support principle in the TISS model context can relate to a practitioner's ability to include peer support in their support team. In practice this could be the formal inclusion of a peer mentor where the purpose and scope are defined within the support team framework. Peer support could also be included in an informal capacity. Informal peer support could be included in a practitioner's support plan as a strategy for practitioners to utilise when they feel this kind of support would be beneficial rather than in a prescribed schedule.

Collaboration and mutuality: The collaboration and mutuality principle can relate to the partnership element central to the TISS framework. The TISS framework holds the practitioner as an equal member within their own TISS team with the ability to define goals and design the steps to achieve those goals. Power constructs and how they may impede a practitioner's ability to fully participate in their own TISS team must be kept on the TISS team's agenda and reviewed regularly.

Empowerment, voice and choice: The empowerment, voice and choice principle in the context of the TISS model relates to a practitioner's ability to name what supports they require to effectively undertake their role. Practitioners may need to be empowered to voice what they need. TISS teams may need to provide examples of what more experienced practitioners have included in their TISS plans. This element has a strong emphasis on the integration of lived experience. In the context of the TISS model, integration of lived experience present within this principle refers to the lived experience of the practitioners themselves, which should always strongly inform individualised TISS plans. Practitioners need to be supported to add or subtract supports as individual circumstances change.

Cultural, historical and gender considerations: The cultural, historical and gender considerations principle in the context of the TISS model can refer to the inclusion of sources of support that a practitioner identifies with. As an example, a female-identifying practitioner may wish to receive supports from other female-identifying professionals. This may be to reduce interruption from patriarchal oppression (real or perceived) and creates an opportunity for a practitioner to engage more fully with their supports. Similarly, a practitioner may wish to engage in supports with another practitioner of the same cultural or language background, again to remove barriers to participation and increase the effectiveness of supports. I have shared throughout the book my own research findings relating to the support and supervision needs of First Nations practitioners who work with vulnerable children and their families. A key learning from this research is not to assume what the support needs of First Nations practitioners might be given the negative experiences First Nations communities have had with child protection authorities. The needs of the practitioner are central in the application of the TISS model. Autonomy over voicing individual need is paramount and assumptions should not be made by line supervisors or managers about what support might best suit individual practitioners.

When looking at the six trauma informed principles in the context of the TISS model, one central theme stands out: the importance of TISS plans being driven by the individual practitioners themselves. It is critical that a practitioner be supported to be an active and equal member of their own TISS team.

Central acknowledgements inherent within the TISS model

In addition to the core principles informing the TISS model, there are a number of additional acknowledgements that are critical to understand when working within the TISS context. I will now discuss those key acknowledgements.

The experience of occupational trauma is an occupational inevitability: Working with vulnerable children and their families exposes practitioners to a level of occupational trauma that is unavoidable. Exposure to occupational trauma can result in occupational traumatic stress, as discussed throughout this book. The experience of occupational traumatic stress is an indication that a practitioner has been exposed to occupational trauma, a normal response to abnormal circumstances. The TISS model acknowledges this reality without qualification.

A practitioner's professional development and wellbeing support cannot be solely managed by their line supervisor or manager: Working with vulnerable children and their families is a complex and highly skilled vocation that is undertaken in trauma-laden practice environments. A practitioner's repeated exposure to trauma is an occupational inevitability. Additionally, a practitioner's knowledge needs to stretch over a myriad of areas, including the causes and presentation of child abuse and neglect, child development, highly developed risk assessment knowledge and skill, interventions that will increase a child's safety within their family of origin and the legislation that guides practice with children in individual jurisdictions, just to skim the surface. It is not feasible, or in my view possible, for an individual line supervisor or manager to provide the quality professional development opportunities needed to develop highly experienced child welfare practitioners in isolation. Additionally, given the nature of occupational traumatic stress and how symptomology can present, there are practical but also ethical considerations that need to be taken into account if the only source of wellbeing support available to practitioners is via their line supervisor or manager.

A practitioner's professional support needs will change over time: A practitioner's support needs will be fluid and change over time. Regular reviews need to be built into a practitioner's TISS plan. TISS plans also need to be flexible and responsive to emerging need, the impetus of which might be a critical incident, as an example. Acknowledging with practitioners that there is an expectation that their needs will change over time facilitates an environment where practitioners have the safety to discuss their current needs as well as what their future needs might be.

Core pillars of the TISS model

Now that we have explored the core principles and central acknowledgements underpinning the TISS model, I will outline the four central pillars that underpin the TISS model. The central pillars are the practitioner, the support team, the organisation and local contextualisation. The TISS model is designed to respond to the individual needs of practitioners while also acknowledging the unique context in which they undertake work with vulnerable children and their families. I will now discuss each pillar in the context of the TISS model.

Practitioners

Practitioners are at the centre of the TISS model. Practitioners come to this kind of work for a myriad of reasons, including that they themselves may have experienced similar trauma to the vulnerable children and their families that they work with. Vulnerable children and their families need healthy and grounded professionals to assist them to navigate through their own trauma and related situational crises and into a space where children's care and protection needs can be met adequately. Practitioners need to be engaged in conversations about their motivations to undertake this kind of work. Within an individual's motivations will be clues that inform what kinds of supports may assist them when they start to inevitably experience the effects of occupational traumatic stress. Anchoring practitioners to the core reasons they chose to undertake work with vulnerable children and their families can be a strategy to move practitioners through their experience of occupational traumatic stress back to a place of internal safety. It may be useful for practitioners to explore what their triggers might be and how they have successfully navigated distressing experiences in the past. It must be acknowledged that there may be ethical considerations about whether or not it is appropriate for a practitioner's line supervisor or manager to engage practitioners in these kinds of conversations. These explorations may be better undertaken between a practitioner and an external supervisor, so that the practitioner feels comfortable discussing their professional support needs without the threat (real or perceived) of such information being used for purposes it wasn't intended for, like performance management or other matters related to a practitioner's conduct.

Another element central to the practitioner pillar is to thoroughly explore the professional background of a practitioner. Many practitioners will come to their roles with varied professional experience inclusive of skills, knowledge and professional interests. Again, these elements of a practitioner's background may give insights into how best to move practitioners through occupational traumatic stress, increasing their feelings of job satisfaction and intention to remain in their position.

It is always preferable to explore these elements when a practitioner is not experiencing acute occupational traumatic stress. While setting up a successful TISS plan in line with the TISS model can be resource intensive in the beginning, establishing these elements at the beginning of a professional relationship will create less stress later for all involved.

TISS team – line supervisors and others

The role of line supervisors, managers and other professional supports are key in the TISS model. Similar to the practitioner pillar, line managers, supervisors and others involved in a practitioner's TISS team will also have a myriad of motivations for undertaking their role in the context of working with vulnerable children and their families. As already outlined, transparency is a core principle informing the TISS model. Therefore, those participating in the model will need to thoroughly reflect on how much information about themselves they are willing to contribute. There is power in expressing vulnerability to those one supervises, especially in relation to motivations for undertaking the work and the strategies one may have used previously to move through the experience of occupational traumatic stress. However, drawing on the work of George Kohlrieser on secure base leadership outlined in the previous chapter, leaders who operate from an internal state of safety are the most effective in guiding practitioners through occupational traumatic stress. Another key principle of the TISS model is critical reflection. It is this principle that calls on all practitioners who make up a TISS team to critically reflect on their own histories of trauma, including their experience of occupational trauma, and to establish where their boundaries are in the context of working within the TISS framework. Protective professional boundaries do not exclude line supervisors, managers and others from participating in the TISS framework. As already outlined, a central acknowledgement underpinning the TISS model is that a practitioner's professional development and wellbeing support cannot be provided by one source. Therefore, if a practitioner feels that their professional development and wellbeing support would benefit from engagement with a professional who at that point in time would be comfortable using their lived experience as a support strategy, then the TISS model allows for this. A team approach to supporting practitioners who work with vulnerable children and their families facilitates the opportunity for practitioners to receive the support they require without compromising the boundaries of line supervisors and managers.

Organisation and local contextualisation

The next two pillars, namely organisations and local contextualisation, are core to the TISS model. They are also the elements that are almost always excluded from practitioner support and supervision plans.

Organisations

Already established in this book is the struggle organisations have had, and continue to have, in providing adequate support and supervision to practitioners that meets their needs. I am not of the view that organisations set out with an explicit agenda to fail their practitioners in this regard. As discussed throughout this book, organisations struggle to provide effective and responsive support to practitioners for numerous complex and intersecting reasons. Acknowledging with practitioners where they are located within a larger system can assist practitioners to work through occupational distress that is rooted in a systemic context. An example of this might be when practitioners develop a sense of hopelessness because they are working within the 'system'. In my own time working with practitioners, it is almost always the 'system' that contributes to a practitioner's decision to leave their role working with vulnerable children and their families rather than the vulnerable children and families themselves. Internalised hopelessness and the feeling that the work practitioners do is meaningless can be overwhelming. This paralysis can lead to practitioners not fully engaging in their work or monitoring their own wellbeing. When a practitioner has a solid understanding of the 'system' in which they work, including from sociological, political and cultural viewpoints, they are in a better professional position to navigate that system and to broker better outcomes for the vulnerable children and their families that they work with. Supporting practitioners to externalise their feelings of hopelessness is an effective strategy for line supervisors and managers attempting to move practitioners through identified occupational traumatic stress.

The TISS model seeks to acknowledge the inherent complexities, including structural, that come with working with vulnerable children and their families. The TISS model seeks to identify these complexities so that mitigation strategies can be included within a practitioner's TISS plan. An example of this might be acknowledging organisational complexities pertaining to practitioner workloads. In most jurisdictions and practice settings, there are policy and procedural guides outlining expectations in relation to workload, especially when it comes to the number of cases an individual practitioner may have responsibility for. However, anyone who has worked in a child welfare organisation knows that there can be a chasm between ideal workloads and the reality. Child welfare organisations are plagued by high staff turnover rates and difficulty recruiting and retaining experienced practitioners, especially in rural and remote communities. High turnover rates contribute to high workloads for the remaining practitioners and their line supervisors and managers. These complexities are reported consistently in the research literature across jurisdictions (Hunt et al., 2016; Oates, 2019). Given the research literature, one can accurately conclude that unreasonable workloads in a child welfare organisation do significantly negatively affect the wellbeing of practitioners. This must be acknowledged in TISS plans. The power of acknowledgement cannot be underestimated. It gives practitioners the safety to raise issues pertaining to workload without the fear of being deemed as not suitable for the position if they cannot keep up with the workload. Strategies may include that workload is added as a standing agenda item in TISS plans and that purposeful, targeted discussions pertaining to workloads occur regularly.

Local contextualisation

Implementing the TISS model without due consideration of matters pertaining to local contextualisation would likely result in less effective results for practitioners. Any practitioner who has worked with vulnerable children and their families in a rural or remote community, or in a community where the dominant culture is not their own, already has an innate understanding of why incorporating local contextualisation into a practitioner's TISS plan is critically important. Having a good understanding of the sociological, economic and political factors that affect communities is invaluable information for practitioners to acquire. Understanding these elements, and being able to analyse community issues from this framework, is a strategy that will facilitate a practitioner's ability to externalise some of the occupational traumatic stress they may experience as a result of working with vulnerable children and their families. There are complex reasons, far bigger than any one individual practitioner, that contribute to children experiencing abuse and neglect. Having said that, practitioners still have a responsibility to undertake professional learning and development to ensure that they have up-to-date knowledge and skills to assist families and communities to best meet the care and protection needs of their children. This is a balance that requires ongoing analysis and evaluation in a supervision context. Questions that a practitioner and their supports may ask themselves within a local context might include:

- What is the history of the community we work in? Does the community have a history of traumatic events like ongoing military conflict, natural disasters, dispossession of land due to colonisation or high rates of humanitarian settlement?
- What is the demographic landscape of the community? Does the community have a lot of older people in comparison to younger people and families, as an example? Are there large numbers of migrant or newly arrived people who don't speak English as a first language?
- What socioeconomic factors affect the community? Is the community categorised as predominantly low in socioeconomic status? What are the unemployment rates? Is there adequate access to housing, education, health care and other social support services? Is there an above average incarceration rate?

Another element of the local contextualisation pillar in the TISS model that requires addressing is how living in the community a practitioner works in affects or potentially affects them. The nature of the work means that working with people that are hostile towards practitioners in this field is inevitable. As an example, the smaller the community you work in, the more likely it is that practitioners are interacting with the vulnerable children and families they work with outside of their regular work hours. Examples of this include attending the same church or social group, having children who attend the same school, who are in the same friendship group or who are on the same sports team. There may only be a handful of shops to purchase groceries, fuel or other essentials. The smaller the community, the more a practitioner's visibility increases. This can lead to practitioners feeling they have to alter how they normally spend their time outside of work, where they go or whom they interact with. Practitioners in my own research stated that they had increased visibility in the communities where they worked due to their Indigeneity, which brings with it a number of complexities. Increased visibility in general can contribute to practitioners not being able to have restful breaks from their work. The other element to keep in mind in the context of this pillar is that the smaller the community, the less access practitioners will have to professionals who may support them with their own issues pertaining to wellbeing. Practitioners may not be comfortable working with a psychologist, social worker or other therapeutic practitioner whom they also interact with on a professional level. This pillar advocates for other options to be explored, like connecting with therapeutic support via phone or video sessions.

The TISS framework

Figure 4.1 is a visual representation of the TISS framework.

Using the TISS model to create TISS teams

Central to the TISS model is the creation of a TISS team around practitioners. An increasingly common approach to managing clients with complex needs in a practice context is the creation of 'care teams'. Care teams are usually established around complex clients and families in acknowledgement that no one organisation or intervention could ever meet all identified needs and that a mixture of professional skills, knowledge, experience and resources is required to meet those needs. Needs are assessed and interventions planned and evaluated by way of a common 'care plan'. The care team model will be familiar to many working with vulnerable children and their families. Pre-existing knowledge of the creation of care teams to meet complex needs within the child welfare sector adds to the transferability of the model to supporting the professional and wellbeing needs of practitioners.

Benefits of implementing a TISS team model

Already identified in this book is the established link between trust in the supervisory relationship and a practitioner's sense of being supported in their place of work. However, it is also true that in a sector

	Core Pillars			
	Practitioner	Supervisor	Organisation	Local Context
The practitioner is central to the TISS model	What are your qualifications? Your professional skills & experiences?	What is the supervisors role? Are they responsible for line supervision? Professional and/or practice supervision? Management of case loads & performance?	How does the organisational context you work in impact your work with vulnerable children & families?	What is the history of the community we work in?
	What do you need from your supervisory relationship?		Statutory vs non-statutory?	Does the community have a history of traumatic events like ongoing military conflict, natural disasters, dispossession of land due to colonisation or high rates of humanitarian settlement?
	What are your professional development needs?	What do supervisors need to provide for the professional development & wellbeing needs of practitioners?	Public, not for profit, for profit?	
Occupational trauma is an occupational inevitability	What are your wellbeing needs?		Sociological, political, cultural factors?	What is the demographic landscape of the community?
	What are your indicators of occupational traumatic stress? What strategies have been successful previously?	Are there gaps in knowledge, skills or experiences that could be filled by others?	Practice or resource restrictions?	What socioeconomic factors impact the community?

Professional development & wellbeing support cannot be met by one source

A practitioner's professional needs will change over time

trauma-informed principles: safety, trustworthiness & transparency; peer support; collaboration & mutuality; empowerment, voice & choice; cultural, historical & gender considerations

Figure 4.1 TISS framework

with such high turnover numbers, an expectation that practitioners and supervisors have long-standing relationships or that trust is something easily established would be naïve. This is where the idea of support teams for practitioners is useful. As an example, if a practitioner is new to a team and has not yet established a relationship with their supervisor that is characterised by a sense of trust and safety, this element could be secured in another way, by another professional in the support team – perhaps a member that does not have line supervisory responsibly for the practitioner. Similarly, if a practitioner feels that professional support provided by someone of the same gender, sexuality, cultural or religious background as themselves would be beneficial, this could be supported within a practitioner's TISS team. Within the literature it has been established that there is a barrier between practitioners seeking assistance from their line supervisors and managers when they are experiencing symptomology of occupational traumatic stress for fear of being viewed as incompetent or not suitable to undertake child protection work (Hunt et al., 2016; Oates, 2019). Having a TISS team provides practitioners with a number of avenues to seek required support without these fears as an impediment.

A team approach to supporting both a practitioner's professional development and wellbeing needs is also beneficial for line supervisors and managers. If a line supervisor or manager starts to struggle with symptoms of occupational traumatic stress themselves, they can move elements of practitioner support for which they are responsible to other members of the TISS team, even if only temporarily. In this example, the flexibility within the TISS model would create space for a line supervisor or manager to resolve their own problematic occupational stress presentations without compromising support available to individual practitioners. Again, a professionally mature acknowledgement of occupational traumatic stress as an occupational inevitability facilitates the ability of practitioners, supervisors and organisations to proactively plan for issues when they arise. Proactive planning is a strategy that will assist in stopping the 'knock on effect' discussed previously, that is, case workers not receiving effective supervision because their line supervisors are struggling, line supervisors not receiving effective supervision because their managers are struggling and so on and so forth. Another scenario for line supervisors and managers where the implementation of the TISS model is useful would be when their own workload becomes difficult to manage. The scenario where support to practitioners is compromised because line supervisors are consistently pulled in other urgent directions is reported repeatedly in the literature by both practitioners and supervisors.

Roles within a practitioner support team

As mentioned previously, a lack of trust and clarity of role and purpose within supervision are identified as threats to a positive supervisory experience in the research literature. Transparency of role and purpose within a practitioner's support team is critical and should be thoroughly discussed and formally documented as a routine part of developing a support plan with a practitioner. The key roles within a practitioner's support team underpinned by the TISS model, namely the practitioner, the line supervisor or manager and additional roles, will now be discussed.

<u>Practitioner:</u> The central role within a practitioner's TISS team is the practitioner themselves. Practitioners must have a sense of ownership of their TISS plan. TISS plans are unique to the individual practitioner and are designed to meet their individual needs. Having said that, practitioners must be active contributors for the model to be successful. Practitioners need to come to the TISS model with an open mind, professional maturity and a clear understanding of what their role is. Practitioners also need to be cognisant of what their responsibilities are as part of the model. For example, if it is the role of the line supervisor to oversee a practitioner's cases, then practitioners need to engage in this process as part of their role. An increased focus on wellbeing in supervision does not exclude a line supervisor or manager discussing performance, conduct issues or practice concerns with practitioners. As with all things, balance is needed.

<u>Line supervisor/manager:</u> A practitioner's line supervisor or manager will play a number of roles within a practitioner's TISS team. The role of the line supervisor or manager will be heavily influenced by a number of factors which might include organisational context (statutory vs non-statutory), professional background of the line supervisor or stipulations related to program funding. Most line supervisors and managers will have the responsibility of managing a practitioner's workload, procedural compliance and other HR matters. These core responsibilities will remain the same in the context of the TISS model. A large proportion of line supervisors and managers will also have the sole responsibility for managing the support and supervision needs of practitioners. Organisationally, that responsibility may be inflexible; however, the TISS model has enough flexibility to ensure that the needs of the organisation are met as well as the needs of the practitioner. A core role of the line supervisor or manager as part of the TISS model is to actively support and encourage practitioners to engage fully in the model. Similarly, line supervisors and managers

must themselves be actively engaged in the model for the implementation to be successful.

Others: As outlined, a core component of the TISS model is the creation of TISS teams around practitioners. Who is on a practitioner's TISS team, in addition to the practitioner and the line supervisor, is a process of negotiation. As with the role of the line manager and supervisor outlined earlier, contextual factors must be considered. Some of these factors may include the payment of external professional supports, funds to pay for professional journal subscriptions or the amount of time allocated to attend sessions, and whether attending during paid work time is acceptable. It might be useful for line supervisors and managers to voice during these negotiations what might be useful for them to best support the needs of individual practitioners. An example might be a practitioner struggling with writing and/or maintaining electronic case notes. A solution might be to link that practitioner with a more experienced practitioner who may act as a mentor, rather than having the line supervisor responsible for all aspects of a practitioner's professional skill development. Other professionals that may be involved in a TISS team might include a professional external supervisor, an internal experienced member of a practitioner's organisation that doesn't have line manager responsibility for said practitioner or professional peers, either individuals or in a group.

Creating a TISS plan with practitioners

For the TISS model to be successful, a number of elements need to be included. As outlined in the research literature, internal supervision with a practitioner's line supervisor or manager that is predominantly administrative in nature seldom meets the needs of practitioners. The TISS model seeks to identify and plan for these research-informed factors so that practitioners have the best opportunity to receive support and supervision that meets both their professional development and wellbeing needs.

Preventative and mitigation factors in TISS plans

Two key elements are identified repeatedly in the research literature that, if present, reduce the impact of occupational traumatic stress on practitioners that work in trauma-laden environments. Those two elements are the experience of job satisfaction and an effective supervisory relationship. When crafting a TISS plan with practitioners, it is important to explicitly explore these factors and to incorporate them formally. I will now explore both of these elements in the context of the TISS framework.

Protective factor: job satisfaction

The experience of job satisfaction was repeatedly referred to in the research literature (Beddoe et al., 2014; Berger & Quiros, 2016; Hunt et al., 2016; Regehr, 2018) as a key protective factor against the problematic experience of occupational trauma. Exploring with a practitioner what elements would elicit a feeling of job satisfaction for them is a critical part of TISS planning. As an example, a practitioner might say that they have experienced the most vivid feeling of job satisfaction when they see children and young people who have experienced abuse and neglect achieve at school. For this practitioner, a job satisfaction element included in their TISS planning might be that they attend school-based activities of the children they are working with, like school plays or sporting events. Another example might be regularly scheduling time with children they are working with when they receive end-of-term reports for the express purpose of celebrating achievement.

Being provided with professional development opportunities was also cited in the literature as a factor increasing practitioner experience of job satisfaction. It might be appropriate to explore with the practitioner, as part of their TISS planning, the kinds of professional development opportunities they might be interested in. It could be attendance at non-compulsory in-house training sessions, attendance at conferences, participation in workshops to learn a new skill or increase knowledge, a subscription to a relevant journal or access to an expert in the field they are interested in. The practitioner then may be asked to contribute a short presentation to the team, who in turn may view the practitioner as a source of knowledge on the topic.

Practical application of the job satisfaction element in workgroups

As with many intervention models, it can be difficult to visualise their application in real-life practice scenarios. I will now explore three examples of what incorporating the element of job satisfaction within a wider workgroup context might look like.

Celebration of successes: Job satisfaction has been clearly established in the literature as a critical factor that contributes positively to practitioner wellbeing. A threat to a practitioner's feelings of job satisfaction includes repetitive tasks without successful outcomes challenging internal dialogue that no difference is being made despite efforts, performing difficult or new tasks that challenge feelings of competency and sustained periods of chaotic work environments with limited predictability. Unfortunately, these threats often characterise the nature of working with vulnerable children and their families regardless of practice setting. Integrating the celebration of successes, however small, can be as straightforward as quarantining a small period of time during formal supervision, or could be more creative and involve others, like a monthly morning tea where celebrations are shared within the staff group.

Job satisfaction focus within teams: In a team context, a strategy to increase team cohesiveness might be for practitioners to share what job satisfaction would look like to them and to share how they centre those opportunities in their day-to-day work plans. A strategy like this may increase the feeling of job satisfaction in other practitioners on the team. Teams that have strong focus on achievement function more cohesively, and this translates into better service delivery outcomes. Further, peer support within cohesive teams tends to be stronger and more effective, especially when new practitioners join. There is a correlation between strong psychological safety within teams and decreases in practitioner turnover (Kruzich et al., 2014).

Culture of achievement rather than bonding over trauma: There is a culture within human services workforces where the telling of 'war stories' bonds practitioners together, and at times, with their organisation. While the sharing of difficult experiences is a healthy strategy in managing occupational traumatic stress, forming one's professional identity around it is not. Professional identities that are rooted in the central belief that no one else understands the work we do, we are the most skilled of workers to the exclusion of other practitioners or professions, is limiting and counterproductive. These cultural identities limit practitioner and organisational ability to critically reflect on their own practice and to think outside the box for creative solutions to complex problems on both a client and organisational level. Further, these cultural underpinnings create dichotomies where the strong amongst the team survive – that is, those practitioners who experience the most traumatic events for the longest period without demonstrating outwardly symptoms of occupational traumatic stress. The traits attributed to the 'strong' amongst the group are significant barriers to practitioners seeking assistance when their experience of occupational traumatic stress starts to become disruptive to their

ability to undertake their role. Feelings of belonging are strong moti-
vators to not seek assistance when doing so would separate a practitioner from the emotional support that comes from feeling part of a
successful team.

Protective factor: supervisory relationship

As previously outlined, the second key element identified in the
research literature as a factor leading to a practitioner's ability to successfully manage symptoms of occupational traumatic stress was an
effective supervisory relationship. As explored in previous chapters, a
strong supervisory relationship between practitioners and line supervisors contributes to a practitioner's ability to critically explore and
improve their practice (Little et al., 2018; Radey & Stanley, 2018),
more successfully manage the symptoms of occupational traumatic
stress (Beddoe et al., 2014; Berger & Quiros, 2016; McPherson et al.,
2016), increase feelings of psychological safety (Kruzich et al., 2014),
increase job satisfaction (Hunt et al., 2016; Regehr, 2018) and build
healthy professional resiliency (Beddoe et al., 2014; McFadden, 2020;
Regehr, 2018). As with the job satisfaction example, it may be beneficial to build in factors to a practitioner's TISS plan that strengthen
the supervisory relationship and thus increase the likelihood of practitioners successfully managing occupational traumatic stress. Activities in a TISS plan that strengthen the supervisory relationship might
include scheduled opportunities for live supervision; that is, shadow-
ing line supervisors while they undertake their own duties. This might
include attending client meetings, meetings with stakeholders or senior members of the organisation where appropriate.

Given the strong evidence that a positive supervisory relationship is
a key contributing factor to maintaining the wellbeing needs of practitioners, explicitly exploring threats to the supervisory relationship is
key within the TISS model. Supervision can elicit uncomfortable feelings for practitioners, particularly if challenging conversations about
clients or their own performance are being discussed. Practitioners
being challenged to critically reflect on their practice is a necessary
and healthy part of any commitment to professional development.
However, managing these uncomfortable feelings in an upfront,
professionally mature way can mitigate threats to the overall supervisory relationship. Key threats to a successful supervisory relationship identified in the research literature include a lack of consistency,
a perceived lack of commitment of the supervisor to the wellbeing
of the practitioner being supervised and practitioner perception

that supervision is a surveillance tool for performance management. It must be noted that although these three elements are repeatedly listed in the research literature, a useful endeavour would be for supervisors and practitioners to identify what they feel might pose a threat to the supervisory relationship and strategies they feel might mitigate those risks.

Addressing these elements in a practitioner's TISS plan could be achieved in any number of ways. As already outlined, the power of acknowledgement cannot be underestimated. Acknowledging that there will be times when the supervisory relationship is strained and planning for those times is a useful strategy. Examples might include exploring how a practitioner might let their line supervisor know that they need some time to process uncomfortable feelings that emerge from supervision. Another example might be exploring what actions or behaviours a line supervisor or manager would have to demonstrate for a practitioner to feel that they are committed to their professional development and wellbeing. These clear, professionally mature conversations in supervision are critical, particularly when a common symptom of occupational traumatic stress is the inability to interpret interactions with others accurately.

Creating a TISS team around those with line management responsibilities

We have established the benefits of creating TISS teams around practitioners to support both their professional development and wellbeing. The TISS model can also be applied to supporting the professional development and wellbeing of line supervisors and managers. The model is transferrable to any position within an organisation where their core business, even if only in part, is to work with vulnerable children and their families. Of course some elements may be different to reflect differences that are role specific. There may be an increased focus on financial management, policy development or strategic leadership upskilling. However, the core framework of the TISS model would be the same, that is, that the practitioner is at the centre and that they are equal contributors both in their TISS team and to their TISS plan.

Supporting documents

There are three companion documents that will assist in establishing a TISS team and a TISS plan. They are the TISS preparation worksheet, the TISS team agreement and the TISS plan proformas. They can be located in the appendix of this book. They are designed to be generic and used as a guide. Individuals and organisations are encouraged to individualise TISS agreements and plans to suit their circumstances and needs.

Chapter summary

In this chapter I have introduced the TISS framework for supporting both the professional development and wellbeing needs of practitioners who work with vulnerable children and their families. The core trauma informed principles of safety, trustworthiness and transparency, peer support, collaboration and mutuality, empowerment, voice and choice and cultural, historical and gender considerations were discussed in the context of the TISS framework. Acknowledgements that are central to the TISS framework – namely, the experience of occupational trauma is an occupational inevitability; a practitioner's professional development and wellbeing support cannot be solely managed by their line supervisor or manager; and a practitioner's professional support needs will change over time – were outlined and discussed. Also discussed were the central pillars of the TISS model; namely, the practitioner, the supervisor, the organisation and local contextualisation. Finally, using the TISS model to create TISS teams and TISS plans was discussed, and included the roles each member has.

Reflective questions for practice

1. As a practitioner, who would you want on your TISS team and why?
2. As a practitioner, what would you like included in your TISS plan and why?
3. As a line supervisor or manager using the TISS model, what element would you find most useful?

References

Beddoe, L., Davys, A., & Adamson, C. (2014). "Never trust anybody who says 'I don't need supervision': Practitioners" beliefs about social worker resilience. *Practice (Birmingham, England)*, 26(2), 113–130. https://doi.org/10.1080/09503153.2014.896888

Berger, R., & Quiros, L. (2016). Best practices for training trauma informed practitioners: Supervisors' voice. *Traumatology, 22*(2), 145–154. doi:10.1037/trm0000076

Hunt, S., Goddard, C., Cooper, J., Littlechild, B., & Wild, J. (2016). 'If I feel like this, how does the child feel?' Child protection workers, supervision, management and organisational responses to parental violence. *Journal of Social Work Practice, 30*(1), 5–24. doi:10.1080/02650533.2015.1073145

Kruzich, J., Mienko, J., & Courtney, M. (2014). Individual and work group influences on turnover intention among public child welfare workers: The effects of work group psychological safety. *Children and Youth Services Review, 42*, 20–27. https://doi.org/10.1016/j.childyouth.2014.03.005

Little, M., Baker, T., & Jinks, A. (2018). A qualitative evaluation of community nurses' experiences of child safeguarding supervision. *Child Abuse Review, 27*(2), 150–157. http://dx.doi.org/10.1002/car.2493.

McFadden, P. (2020). Two sides of one coin? Relationships build resilience or contribute to burnout in child protection social work: Shared perspectives from leavers and stayers in Northern Ireland. *International Social Work, 63*(2), 164–176. doi:10.1177/0020872818788393

McPherson, L., Frederico, M., & McNamara, P. (2016). Safety as a fifth dimension in supervision: Stories from the frontline. *Australian Social Work, 69*(1), 67–79. doi:10.1080/0312407X.2015.1024265

Oates, F. (2019). You are not allowed to tell: Organisational culture as a barrier for child protection workers seeking assistance for traumatic stress symptomology. *Children Australia, 44*(2), 84–90. doi:10.1017/cha.2019.12

Radey, M., & Stanley, L. (2018). "Hands on" versus "empty": Supervision experiences of frontline child welfare workers. *Children and Youth Services Review, 91*, 128–136. https://doi.org/10.1016/j.childyouth.2018.05.037

Regehr, C. (2018). *Stress, trauma, and decision-making for social workers.* Columbia University Press.

Substance Abuse and Mental Health Services Administration. (2014). *SAMHSA's concept of trauma and guidance for a trauma informed approach.* Substance Abuse and Mental Health Services Administration.

Appendices
Appendix 1.1
TISS preparation worksheet

This worksheet is designed for practitioners to use in preparation for the development of their TISS plan. Below the template are the definitions informing both the trauma informed principles and the core pillars in the context of the TISS framework for reference.

Date: _____

Practitioner name: _____

Practitioner role: _____

Current qualifications: _____

Professional experience: _____

_____

Trauma informed principles	*Examples of how I can be supported in my role*
Safety Trustworthiness and transparency Peer support Collaboration and mutuality Empowerment, voice and choice Cultural, historical and gender considerations	

TISS pillars			
Practitioner	*Supervisor*	*Organisation*	*Local Contextualisation*

TISS preparation worksheet definitions

Trauma informed principles

These are the trauma informed principles that inform the TISS model. Please refer back to these when completing the preparation worksheet.

<u>Safety</u>: The safety principle applied within the TISS model context can refer to apractitioner's sense of safety within the supervisory relationship, both perceived and actual. The literature on practitioner experience of supervision has found that some practitioners avoid engaging in meaningful supervision due to a view that supervision is a tool used by their organisation to surveil them and their work. The safety principle can also underpin a practitioner's decision to share matters pertaining to their wellbeing.

<u>Trustworthiness and transparency</u>: The trustworthiness and transparency principle in the TISS model can refer to a shared sense of trust between a practitioner and their supervisor. As mentioned previously, the building and maintenance of trust in the supervisory relationship is critical and has been identified in the research literature as a key factor in a practitioner's ability to move through traumatic occupational experiences. The transparency part of this element should refer to transparency within the supervision process, that is, having clarity on the purpose of supervision, why certain matters are discussed and what the information will and will not be used for.

<u>Peer support</u>: The peer support principle in the TISS model context can relate to a practitioner's ability to include peer support in their support team. In practice this could be the formal inclusion of a peer mentor where the purpose and scope are defined within the support team framework. Peer support could also be included in a non-formal capacity. Informal peer support could be included in a practitioner's support plan as a strategy for practitioners to utilise when they feel this kind of support would be beneficial rather than in a prescribed schedule.

<u>Collaboration and mutuality</u>: Collaboration and mutuality can relate to the partnership element central to the TISS framework. The TISS framework holds the practitioner as an equal member of their own support team with the ability to define goals and design the steps to achieve those goals. Power constructs and how they may impede a practitioner's ability to fully participate in their own TISS team needs to be kept on the TISS team's agenda and reviewed regularly.

Empowerment, voice and choice: The empowerment, voice and choice principle in the context of the TISS model relates to a practitioner's ability to name what supports they require to effectively undertake their duties. Practitioners may need to be empowered to voice what they need. TISS teams may need to provide examples of what more experienced practitioners have included in their support plans so that visualising possible needs might become clearer. This element has a strong emphasis on the integration of lived experience. In the context of the TISS model, 'integration of lived experience' refers to the lived experience of the practitioner themselves, which should always strongly inform individualised supervision and support plans. Practitioners must be permitted to add or subtract supports as individual circumstances change.

Cultural, historical and gender considerations: The cultural, historical and gender considerations principle in the context of the TISS model can refer to the inclusion of sources of support that a practitioner identifies with. As an example, a female-identifying practitioner may wish to receive support from other female-identifying professionals. This may be to reduce interruption by patriarchal oppression (real or perceived) and creates an opportunity for a practitioner to engage more fully with their supports. Similarly, a practitioner may wish to engage in support with another practitioner of the same cultural or language background, again to remove barriers to participation and increase the effectiveness of supports. I have shared throughout the book my own research findings relating to the support and supervision needs of First Nations practitioners who work with vulnerable children and their families. A key learning from this research is not to assume what the support needs of a First Nations practitioner might be, given the negative historical and current experiences of First Nations communities with regard to child protection authorities. The needs of the practitioner are central in the application of the TISS model. Autonomy over voicing individual need is paramount and assumptions should not be made by line supervisors or managers about what support might best suit individual practitioners.

Core pillars

There are four pillars that support the TISS framework. They are the practitioner, the supervisor, the organisation and local contextualisation. The four pillars of the TISS framework are further defined as follows. Please refer to them when completing this worksheet.

Practitioners: Practitioners are at the centre of the TISS model. Practitioners come to this kind of work for a myriad of reasons, including that they themselves may have experienced similar trauma to the vulnerable children and their families whom they work with. Vulnerable children and their families need healthy and grounded professionals to assist them to navigate through their own trauma and related situational crises and into a space where children's care and protection needs are met adequately. Practitioners need to be engaged in conversations about their motivations to undertake this kind of work. Within an individual's motivations will be clues that inform what kinds of supports may assist them when they start to inevitably experience the effects of occupational traumatic stress. Anchoring practitioners to the core reasons they chose to undertake work with vulnerable children and their families can be a strategy to move practitioners through their experience of occupational traumatic stress back to a place of internal safety. It may be useful for practitioners to explore what their triggers might be and how they have successfully navigated distressing experiences in the past. It must be acknowledged that there may be ethical considerations about whether or not it is appropriate for a practitioner's line supervisor or manager to engage practitioners in these kinds of conversations. These explorations may be better undertaken between a practitioner and an external supervisor, so that the practitioner feels comfortable discussing their professional support needs without the threat (real or perceived) of such information being used for purposes it wasn't intended for, like performance management or other matters related to a practitioner's conduct.

Another element central to the practitioner pillar is to thoroughly explore the professional background of a practitioner. Many practitioners come to their roles with varied professional experience inclusive of skills, knowledge and professional interests. Again, these elements of a practitioner's background may give insights into how best to move practitioners through occupational traumatic stress, increasing their feelings of job satisfaction and intention to remain in their position.

It is always preferable to explore these elements when a practitioner is not experiencing acute occupational traumatic stress. While setting up a successful TISS plan in line with the TISS model can be resource intensive in the beginning, having these elements established at the beginning of a professional relationship will create less stress for all involved later.

TISS team – line supervisors and others: The role of line supervisors, managers and other professional supports are key in the context of the TISS model. Similar to the practitioner pillar, line managers, supervisors and others involved in a practitioner's TISS team will also have many motivations for undertaking the role that they do in the context of working with vulnerable children and their families. As already outlined, transparency is a core principle informing the TISS model. Therefore, those participating in the model will need to thoroughly reflect on how much information about themselves they are willing to contribute. There is power in expressing vulnerability to those one supervises, especially in relation to motivations for undertaking the work and the strategies one may have used previously to move through the experience of occupational traumatic stress. However, drawing on the work of George Kohlrieser on secure base leadership outlined earlier, leaders who operate from an internal state of safety are the most effective in guiding practitioners through occupational traumatic stress. Another key principle of the TISS model is critical reflection. It is this principle that calls on all practitioners who make up a TISS team to critically reflect on their own histories of trauma, including their experience of occupational trauma, and to establish where their boundaries are in the context of the TISS framework. Protective professional boundaries do not exclude line supervisors, managers and others from participating in the TISS framework. As already outlined, a central acknowledgement underpinning the TISS model is that a practitioner's professional development and wellbeing support cannot be provided by one source. Therefore, if a practitioner feels that their professional development and wellbeing support would benefit from engagement with a professional who at that point in time would be comfortable using their lived experience as a support strategy, then the TISS model allows for this. A team approach to supporting practitioners who work with vulnerable children and their families facilitates the opportunity for practitioners to receive the support they require without compromising the boundaries of line supervisors and managers.

Organisation: Already established in this book is the struggle organisations have had, and continue to have, in providing adequate support and supervision to practitioners that meets their needs. I am not of the view that organisations set out with an explicit agenda to fail their practitioners in this regard. As discussed throughout this book, organisations struggle to provide effective and responsive support to practitioners for numerous complex and intersecting reasons. Acknowledging with practitioners where they are located within a larger system can assist practitioners to work through occupational distress that is rooted in a systemic context. An example of this might be when practitioners develop a sense of hopelessness because they are working within the 'system'. In my own time working with practitioners, it is almost always the 'system' that contributes to a practitioner's decision to leave their role working with vulnerable children and their families rather than the vulnerable children and families themselves. Internalised hopelessness and the feeling that the work practitioners do is meaningless can be overwhelming. This paralysis can lead to practitioners not fully engaging in their work or monitoring their own wellbeing. When a practitioner has a solid understanding of the 'system' in which they work, including from a sociological, political and cultural viewpoint, they are in a better professional position to navigate that system and to broker better outcomes for the vulnerable children and their families whom they work with. Supporting practitioners to externalise their feelings of hopelessness is an effective strategy for line supervisors and managers attempting to move practitioners through identified occupational traumatic stress.

The TISS model seeks to acknowledge the inherent complexities, including structural, that come with working with vulnerable children and their families. The TISS model seeks to identify these complexities so that mitigation strategies can be included within a practitioner's TISS plan. An example of this might be acknowledging organisational complexities pertaining to practitioner workloads. In most jurisdictions and practice settings, there are policy and procedural guides outlining expectations in relation to workload, especially when it comes to the number of cases an individual practitioner may have responsibility for. However, anyone who has worked in a child welfare organisation knows that there can be a chasm between ideal workloads and reality. Child welfare organisations are plagued by high staff turnover rates and difficulty recruiting and retaining experienced practitioners, especially in rural and remote communities. High turnover rates contribute to high workloads for the remaining practitioners and their line supervisors and managers. These complexities are reported consistently in the research literature across jurisdictions (Hunt et al., 2016; Oates, 2019). Given the research literature, one can accurately conclude that unreasonable workloads within a child welfare organisational context do significantly negatively affect the wellbeing of practitioners and must be acknowledged within TISS plans. The power of acknowledgement cannot be underestimated. It will give practitioners the safety to raise issues pertaining to workload without the fear of being deemed as not suitable for the position if they cannot keep up with the workload. Strategies may include that workload is added as a standing agenda item in TISS plans and that purposeful targeted discussions pertaining to workloads occur regularly.

Local contextualisation: Implementing the TISS model without due consideration of matters pertaining to local contextualisation would likely result in less effective results for practitioners. Any practitioner who has worked with vulnerable children and their families in a rural or remote community, or in a community where the dominant culture is not their own, already has an innate understanding of why incorporating local contextualisation into a practitioner's TISS plan is critically important. Having a good understanding of the sociological, economic and political factors that affect communities is invaluable information for practitioners to acquire. Understanding these elements, and being able to analyse community issues from this framework, is a strategy that facilitates a practitioner's ability to externalise some the occupational traumatic stress they may experience as a result of working with vulnerable children and their families. There are complex reasons, far bigger than any one individual practitioner, that contribute to children experiencing abuse and neglect. Having said that, practitioners still have a responsibility to undertake professional learning and development to ensure that they have up-to-date knowledge and skills to assist families and communities to best meet the care and protection needs of their children. This is a balance that requires ongoing analysis and evaluation in a supervision context. Questions that a practitioner and their supports may ask themselves within a local contextualisation might include:

- What is the history of the community we work in? Does the community have a history of traumatic events like ongoing military conflict, natural disasters, dispossession of land due to colonisation or high rates of humanitarian settlement?
- What is the demographic landscape of the community? Does the community have a lot of older people in comparison to younger people and families, as an example? Are there large numbers of migrant or newly arrived people who don't speak English as a first language?
- What socioeconomic factors impact the community? Is the community categorised as predominantly low in socioeconomic status? Is there adequate access to housing, education, health care and other social support services? Is there an above average incarceration rate?

Another element of the local contextualisation pillar within the TISS model that requires addressing is how living in the community a practitioner works in affects or could potentially affect them. The nature of the work means that working with people who are hostile towards practitioners in this field is inevitable. As an example, the smaller the community you work in, the more likely it is that practitioners are interacting with the vulnerable children and families they work with outside their regular work hours. Examples of this include attending the same church or social group, having children who attend the same school, who are in the same friendship group or who are on the same sports team. There may only be a handful of shops to purchase groceries, fuel or other essentials. The smaller the community, the more a practitioner's visibility increases. This can lead to practitioners feeling they have to alter how they normally spend their time outside of work, where they go or whom they interact with. Practitioners in my own research stated that they had increased visibility within the community they worked due to their Indigeneity, which brings with it a number of complexities. Increased visibility in general can contribute to practitioners not being able to have restful breaks from their work. The other element to keep in mind in the context of this pillar is that the smaller the community, the less access practitioners will have to professionals who may support them with their own issues pertaining to wellbeing. Practitioners may not be comfortable working with a psychologist, social worker or other therapeutic practitioner whom they also interact with on a professional level. This pillar advocates for other options to be explored, like connecting with therapeutic support via phone or video sessions.

References

Hunt, S., Goddard, C., Cooper, J., Littlechild, B., & Wild, J. (2016). 'If I feel like this, how does the child feel?' Child protection workers, supervision, management and organisational responses to parental violence. *Journal of Social Work Practice, 30*(1), 5–24. doi:10.1080/02650533.2015.1073145

Oates, F. (2019). You are not allowed to tell: Organisational culture as a barrier for child protection workers seeking assistance for traumatic stress symptomology. *Children Australia, 44*(2), 84–90. doi:10.1017/cha.2019.12

Appendix 1.2

TISS team agreement

The TISS team agreement should include the date the agreement was made, a support statement that demonstrates the team's (including the practitioner's) commitment to the TISS process, name and roles of those in the team, the frequency of supports, a communication agreement including how issues or disputes are to be managed, the resource allocation required, the date of review and participant signatures.

Date: _____

Support statement: _____

Practitioner name and role: _____

Supervisor: _____

Others and their role: _____

Frequency: _____

Communication agreement: _____

Resource allocation: _____

Review date: _____

Signatures: _____

Following are some suggestions about how to complete the domains in the proforma:

Date: date the agreement is undertaken

Support statement: a support statement should reflect the TISS team's commitment to the practitioner at the centre of the TISS plan as well as a commitment to the model of support

Practitioner name and role: a practitioner's role (including core duties) should be clearly defined – it might be that a practitioner's position description is used to formulate parts of the plan. If a practitioner's role changes or additional duties are added, the TISS plan will need to be reviewed

Supervisor's name and core role: include name and role within the TISS team

Others and their role: include names and role within the TISS team

Frequency: frequency should include sessions between a practitioner and line supervisor as well as frequency of engagements with others in the TISS plan, like an external supervisor, community of practice group, etc.

Communication agreement: a communication agreement should be developed between all members of the TISS team. Consider what kinds of information should be shared between members. An example might be, what kind of information should be shared between an external supervisor and an internal line supervisor about matters discussed by practitioners in sessions, if any? Consider how best to manage issues or disputes that may arise between members of the TISS team, including the practitioner. Where will information about sessions be recorded, who will have access within the TISS team? How should feedback be given?

Resource allocation: include costs of external providers, journal subscriptions, etc., as well as in-kind costs like sessions attended during work hours. How will additional costs be met – e.g., organisationally or by the practitioner?

Review date: TISS agreements and plans should be reviewed regularly. Review periods should be discussed and agreed upon mutually, as should the conditions that would necessitate an earlier review like a role change, illness or performance issue.

Appendix 1.3
TISS plan

This example TISS plan is to give practitioners, supervisors and others an idea of what should be included in a TISS plan. Individuals and organisations are encouraged to develop their own pro forma documents to suit their operational needs. Information from the preparation worksheet should be included in the TISS plan. This TISS framework should be in the fore of mind when completing the TISS plan.

Date: _____

Practitioner name and role:_____

Supervisor: _____

Others and their role: _____

Current qualifications: _____

Professional experience: _____

_____

Review date: _____

Signatures: _____

Following are some suggestions about how to complete the domains in the pro forma:

Professional development needs: This section pertains to the professional education and development needs of practitioners. Items might include upcoming training, formal mentoring arrangements with line supervisors or other colleagues, journal subscriptions or access to a professional library. This would also be the section to discuss levels of job satisfaction as well as professional aspirations.

Wellbeing needs: The wellbeing section is where a practitioner outlines what their needs are in relation to maintaining their wellbeing in the workplace. Information from the TISS preparation worksheet should be included here.

Organisational needs: This section should include things like workload allocation, case reviews, outputs, completion rates, etc. This is also the section to discuss current organisational demands like staffing rates, current key organisational foci and upcoming changes in policies, procedures or practices.

Administration: The administration section is where things like leave applications, issues pertaining to salary, timesheets, employment conditions, etc., are discussed.

Expectations of the practitioner: This is the section where practitioners should explicitly outline their expectations of their line supervisor. Items that may be included here are frequency of supervision, protocols around cancelling or re-scheduling sessions, behaviour that demonstrates an interest in the practitioner's professional development and wellbeing, preferred form of feedback, the process to raise issues or concerns, reasonable timeframes to receive responses to requests, etc. This section should be informed by the TISS preparation document.

Expectations of the supervisor: This section is where the line supervisor or manager outlines their expectations of the practitioner, including similar items to the practitioner.

Expectations of others involved: Although this section may not be included in all instances, it would include expectations pertaining to other members of the TISS team, for example an external supervisor. An external supervisor may include expectations like cancellation policies, payments, scheduling, information exchange, etc. If a practitioner has a community of practice as part of their TISS team, the community of practice wouldn't be included in this section.

Index

Note: Page numbers in *italic* indicate a figure on the corresponding page.

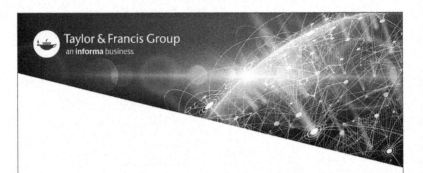

Lightning Source UK Ltd.
Milton Keynes UK
UKHW022023170922
409043UK00010B/95

9 780367 458959